Clinical Pathology
of the
Endocrine Ovary

Clinical Pathology of the Endocrine Ovary

EDITED BY

J. de Brux and J.-P. Gautray

Faculty of Medicine
Université Paris, Val-de-Marne

SPRINGER-SCIENCE+BUSINESS MEDIA, B.V.

Published in the UK and Europe by
MTP Press Limited
Falcon House
Lancaster, England

British Library Cataloguing in Publication Data

Clinical pathology of the endocrine ovary.
1. Ovaries—Diseases   2. Mammals
3. Endocrinology
I. Brux, J. de   II. Gautray, Jean-Pierre
599.02'16   QL881

ISBN 978-94-015-1131-5   ISBN 978-94-015-1129-2 (eBook)
DOI 10.1007/978-94-015-1129-2

Published in the USA by
MTP Press
A division of Kluwer Boston Inc
190 Old Derby Street
Hingham, MA 02043, USA

Library of Congress Cataloging in Publication Data

Main entry under title:

Clinical pathology of the endocrine ovary.

Includes bibliographical references and index.
1. Ovaries—Diseases.   2. Endocrine gynecology.
3. Ovulation.   I. Brux, Jean de.   II. Gautray, Jean-Pierre.
[DNLM: 1. Ovary—Physiology.   2. Ovarian diseases—
Physiopathology.   3. Sex hormones—Physiology.
WP 520 C641]
RG444.C55 1984   618.1'107   84–5666

Phototypeset and
Mather Bros (Printers) Limited, Preston, England

Contents

IV CLINICAL PHYSIOPATHOLOGY

List of Contributors

S. J. ATLAS
Department of Physiology
University of Maryland at Baltimore
School of Medicine
655 W. Redwood Street
Baltimore, MD 21201
USA

M. BENAHMED
INSERM U. 162
Hôpital Debrousse
29 rue Soeur Bouvier
69322 Lyon Cédex 05
France

J. BÉZARD
Physiologie de la Reproduction
INRA, Nouzilly
F-37380 Monnaie
France

F. CABANNE
Centre Georges-François Leclerc
91 rue de Seine
F-75006 Paris
France

C. P. CHANNING
Department of Physiology
University of Maryland at Baltimore
School of Medicine
655 W. Redwood Street
Baltimore, MD 21201
USA

M. C. COLIN
Gynaecology and Obstetrics
Faculté de Médecine de Creteil
CHIC, 40 avenue de Verdun
F-94010 Creteil Cédex
France

J. de BRUX
Institut de Pathologie et de Cytologie
  Appliquée
53/57 rue des Belles Feuilles
B.P. 450-16
F-75769 Paris Cédex 16
France

J.-P. GAUTRAY
Gynaecology and Obstetrics
Faculté de Médecine de Creteil
CHIC, 40 avenue de Verdun
94010 Creteil Cédex
France

C. GOMPEL
Institut Jules Bordet
Centre des Tumeurs de l'Université Libre de
  Bruxelles
1 rue Héger Bordet
B-1000 Bruxelles
Belgium

A. GOUGEON
Physiologie et Psychologie de la Reproduction
  Humaine
INSERM U. 187
32 rue des Carnets
F-92140 Clamart
France

G. D. HODGEN
Pregnancy Research Branch
National Institute of Child Health and Human
  Development
National Institutes of Health
Bethesda, MD 20205
USA

N. KITT
Institut Jules Bordet
Centre des Tumeurs de l'Université Libre de
  Bruxelles
1 rue Héger Bordet
B-1000 Bruxelles
Belgium

A. E. LAMBERT
College de Médecine des Hôpitaux de Paris
11 rue de l'Université
F-75007 Paris
France

M.-J. LEBOUTET
Pathological Anatomy 1—Electron
  Microscopy
CHU Dupuytren
02 avenue Alexis Carrel
F-87042 Limoges Cédex
France

M. R. LOEKEN
Department of Physiology
University of Maryland at Baltimore
School of Medicine
655 W. Redwood Street
Baltimore, MD 21201
USA

A. LOUBET
Pathological Anatomy 1—Electron
  Microscopy
CHU Dupuytren
02 avenue Alexis Carrel
F-87042 Limoges Cédex
France

R. LOUBET
Pathological Anatomy 1—Electron
  Microscopy
CHU Dupuytren
02 avenue Alexis Carrel
F-87042 Limoges Cédex
France

P. MAULEON
Physiologie de la Reproduction
INRA, Nouzilly
F-37380 Monnaie
France

K. NAHOUL
Fondation de Recherche en Hormonologie
67 boulevard Pasteur
94 Fresnes
France

A. P. NETTER
College de Médecine des Hôpitaux de Paris
11 rue de l'Université
F-75007 Paris
France

K. G. OSTEEN
Department of Physiology
University of Maryland at Baltimore
School of Medicine
655 W. Redwood Street
Baltimore, MD 21201
USA

J. REVENTOS
INSERM U. 162
Hôpital Debrousse
29 rue Soeur Bouvier
69322 Lyon Cédex 05
France

J. S. RICHARDS
Cell Biology
Baylor College of Medicine
1200 Moursund Drive
Houston, TX 77030
USA

D. ROTTEN
Gynaecology and Obstetrics
Faculté de Médecine de Creteil
CHIC, 40 avenue de Verdun
F-94010 Creteil Cédex
France

J. M. SAEZ
INSERM U. 162
Hôpital Debrousse
29 rue Soeur Bouvier
69322 Lydon Cédex 05
France

J. C. THALABARD
Gynaecology and Obstetrics
Faculté de Médecine de Creteil
CHIC, 40 avenue de Verdun
F-94010 Creteil Cédex
France

J. P. VIELH
Gynaecology and Obstetrics
Faculté de Médecine de Creteil
CHIC, 40 avenue de Verdun
F-94010 Creteil Cédex
France

I—Embryology

1
The role of mesonephros in ovarian organogenesis

P. Mauleon and J. Bezard

In the mammalian female, the ovigerous cords appear early in the fetal ovary[1]. These cords are constituted by two cellular types: germinal cells (the future oocytes) and somatic cells (the follicular cell precursors).

At sexual differentiation in the male, anatomically defined structures individualize into seminiferous cords. They are delineated by a basal lamina which is seen earlier than ovigerous cords. The seminiferous cords are also composed of germinal cells (the future spermatogonia, spermatocytes and spermatozoa) and somatic cells (the sertoli cell precursors).

The extragonadic origin of the germinal cells has been well established as has their migration to the genital ridge[2]. The origin of somatic elements of the ovigerous and seminiferous cords remains very confused and constitutes one of the unresolved problems in mammalian embryogenesis.

It has often been proposed that these somatic cells originate in the germinal epithelium and that their particular arrangement in the cords results in the different patterns of gametogenesis of the two sexes (ovary and testis). According to this hypothesis, if the genetic sex is a male, germinal epithelium proliferations invade the underlaying mesenchyme where they successively form seminiferous cords and tubules. If the genetic sex is a female, there is initially a proliferation similar to that in the male which forms the medullary cords often described in the ovary centre; then, a second proliferation from the germinal epithelium expands to form the cortical or ovigerous cords. The germinal cells undergo the first phases of the meiotic prophase earlier in the ovigerous cords than in the seminiferous cords.

The histologists of the last century[3-5] mentioned important relationships between the mesonephros and the gonad, and especially these sex cords, in both the male and female. These studies were forgotten until the same observations were made more recently[6,7].

In the ovaries of mice and other species, the primordial follicles maintain some relationship with an extragonadic rete ovarii of mesonephric origin, visible by classic histological techniques (mouse: 13–16 days post-coitum (p.c.) and 7 days post-natal[8]; cat, vison and ferret[9]). These authors suggested that the system

3

of rete cells contributed to the formation of the follicles. This hypothesis was based on very strong evidence but has not been supported by a morphological proof[10].

Reservations about the importance of the role of the mesonephros during gonadal organogenesis have been maintained for a long time because the conclusions come from descriptions of degenerative phenomena in the mesonephric cells of the medullary ovarian area[11]. In recent work, these phenomena have again been described (sheep: 58 days p.c.[12]; macaque: 43 days p.c.[13]).

On reading the old publications we have often been surprised by the audacity of the imagination of these histologists. In fact, their conclusions were based on: observations of incomplete series of embryos of different ages; staining and fixation techniques that did not give clear pictures of the spatial relationships between somatic cells and germinal cells; observation of unoriented sections; and cutting at random in the gonad without the possibility of reconstituting the structures spatially. It was therefore difficult to support their final conclusions on the ovarian and testicular organogenesis[14]. However, we have taken these precautions and are sure the mesonephros has a role in the formation of the primitive sexual cords during organogenesis.

COLONIZATION OF THE GONAD BY THE MESONEPHRIC CELLS (Figure 1)

In the female sheep embryo, *mesonephric cell colonization* of the gonad occurs around days 24–26 of fetal life, at the same time as the early stages of the *giant nephron involution*. The giant nephron is a structure found in the entire cranial third of the mesonephros and consists of a very long, prominent glomerulus in ventral position and a large number of dorsally-situated excretory tubules. It is also present in the mesonephros of the cow and of the deer[15].

The regression of the giant nephron has some unique features: it is accompanied by a massive and sustained mobilization of glomerular and tubular cells which migrate outside the mesonephros, invade the undifferentiated sex gonad and the ovary. Thus, mesangial and epithelial cells move out of the glomerulus, which has no Bowman's capsule, and move into the periglomerular mesenchyme. At this stage, the mesonephric cells have highly irregular profiles which suggests that they migrate towards and into the gonad by amoeboid movement. The mesangial cells are identifiable by their intense affinity for toluidine blue, and the visceral epithelial cells by their numerous, slender microvilli. From day 24 of fetal life, it is possible to follow the colonization of the mesonephric cells outside the glomerulus with these precise cellular markers in thin sections. They migrate from the caudal and ventral giant glomerulus and congregate in small clusters throughout the mesenchyme of the germinal ridge where somatic cell clusters become closely associated with primordial germ cells.

EXISTENCE OF A CONNECTING CORD BETWEEN MESONEPHROS AND GONAD (Figure 2)

The organization of small trabeculae at day 28 and day 29 of the fetal life is followed by formation of a highly compact, cylindrical mass of mesonephric cells. By day 31 (sexual differentiation) this mass extends as a connecting cord

4

from the cranial third of the mesonephros into the ovary. It continues to progress until day 52–58 of the fetal life but its cellular structure changes considerably. By day 60 of the fetal life, the cell mobilization from the residual mesonephric tubules has stopped and the mesonephric cell mass separates from the original nephric structure. This phenomenon is associated with the regression of the giant glomerulus and must be considered together with the sequential stages of ovarian development.

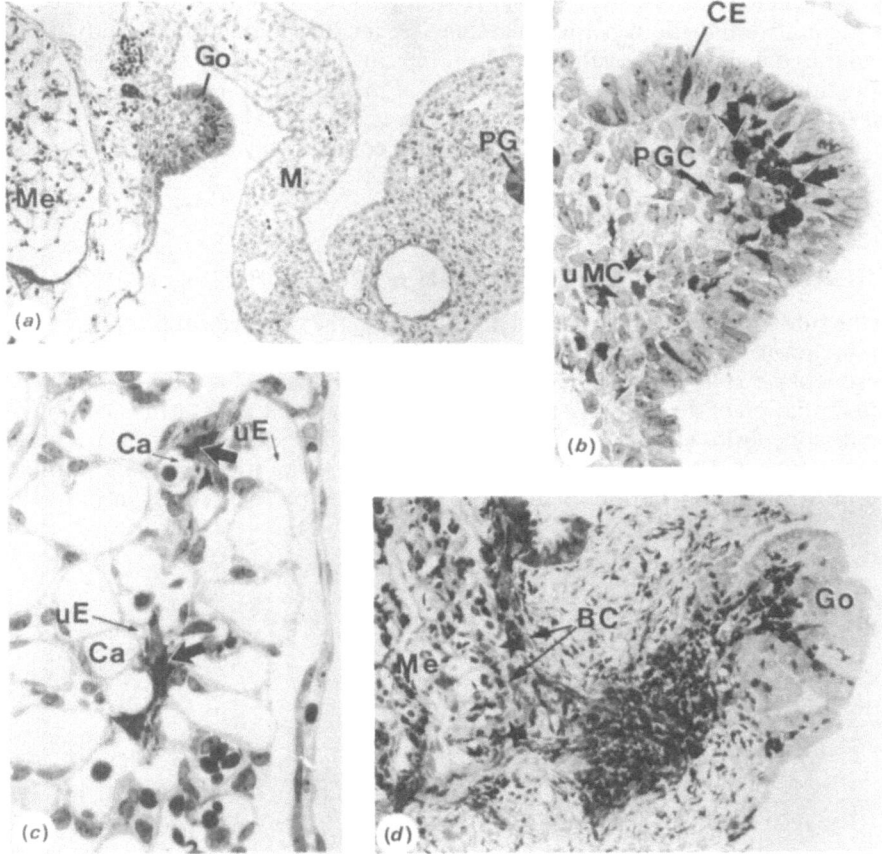

Figure 1 Colonization of the gonad by the mesonephric cells. Cross-sections of sheep embryo, 1 μm thick, stained with toluidine blue. (*a*) In a 24-day-old embryo, germ cells migrate from the primitive gut (PG) by the dorsal mesentery (M) to the gonad (Go) which is only a genital ridge close to the giant glomerulus of the mesonephros (Me) (× 77). (*b*) At high magnification, the gonad is delimited by a layer of mesothelial cells of the coelomic epithelium (CE); it contains undifferentiated mesenchymal cells (uMC), primordial germinal cells (PGC) and a few mesangial cells (broad arrows) of mesonephric origin identifiable from their tinctorial affinity with toluidine blue (× 252). (*c*) Giant glomerulus in a 24-day-old embryo: the mesangial cells (broad arrows) are visible with their high colouration between the very thin capillary walls (Ca) and the visceral epithelial cells running along urinary space (uE) (× 252). (*d*) Early stage of involution of the giant glomerulus (Me) in a 31-day-old embryo. The capillary walls are thickened, the Bowman's capsule (BC) is missing in different areas (★) so glomerular mesangial and epithelial cells egress from the glomerulus (Me) to the gonad (Go) (× 126)

PARALLEL INVOLUTION OF GIANT NEPHRON WITH OVARIAN ORGANIZATION (Figure 2(c) and (d))

The regression of the giant nephron begins around day 24–26 of fetal life. It is initiated in the proximal region and then spreads distally affecting different nephrons at different times. The glomerulus is delineated by a thin capsule of epithelial cells laying on a basal lamina.

From day 28 of the fetal life, the capillary lamina becomes narrower and its walls thicken. In many areas on the ventral part of the glomerulus, the capsule is attenuated and the basal laminae may be missing altogether. By day 34 of fetal life, the giant glomerulus shows all the signs of advanced involution, with reduction of the capillary bed, obliteration of their lumens, fragmentation of the basal laminae with accumulation of collagen and hyalin along the walls. By day 41 of the fetal life, the giant glomerulus is considerably reduced in size and undergoing fibrosis. It has completely regressed by day 52 when only few excretory tubules remain.

ORGANIZATION OF THE OVARIAN STRUCTURE (Figure 3)

In the subsequent stages of ovarian development, the mesonephros appears to be an 'organizer' of the ovary. There is a relationship between the sex cords, where mesonephric cells are very well settled, and the regressing glomerulus. The differentiation of the sex cords starts and follows the same path as the invasion of the mesonephric cells. At the time of the sexual differentiation (day 31), a basal lamina appears near the mesonephros. It is around the trabeculae and around the most proximal portion of the mass resulting from their confluence. In the

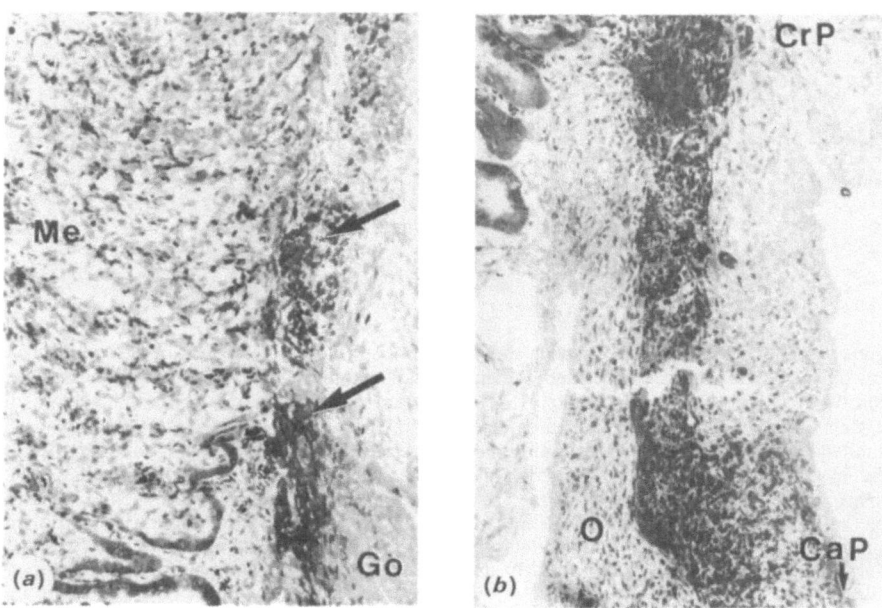

Figure 2

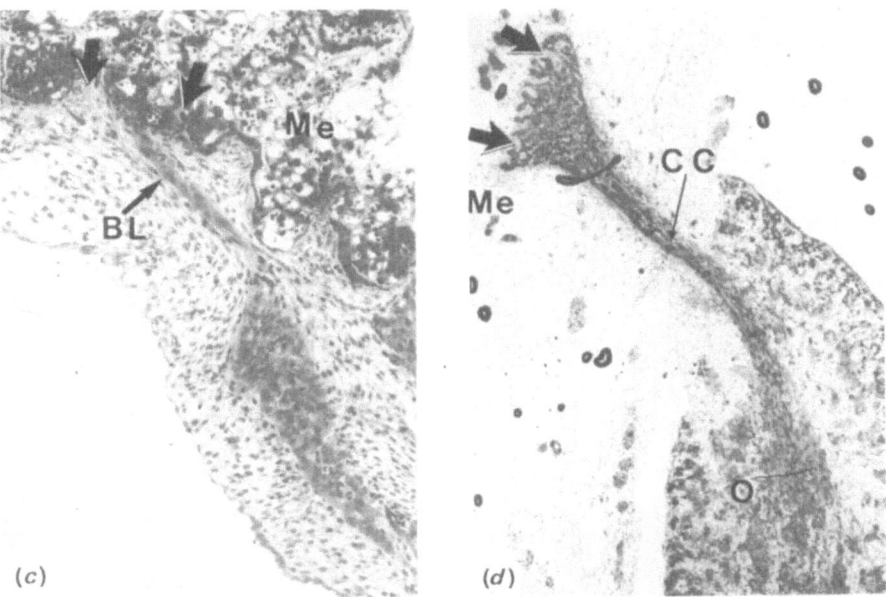

Figure 2 Connecting cord between mesonephros and gonad involution of giant nephron. Longitudinal sections of sheep embryo, 1 μm thick, stained with toluidine blue. (a) In a 28-day-old embryo, glomerular and tubular cell evolution in the cranial part of the mesonephros (Me) form a cellular mass (arrows) migrating to the gonad as yet undifferentiated (Go) (× 88). (b) Female fetus, 34 days old. The dense mesonephric cell mass extends from the giant nephron (not included in the micrograph) into the ovary (O). It progressively becomes less compact from the cranial part (CrP) to the caudal part (CaP). Then this cord is scattered in the gonad and the isolated mesonephric cells establish a close association with the germinal cells (× 88). (c) Female fetus, 41 days old. The cranial part of the compact mesonephric cell mass surrounded by a basal lamina (BL) departs from giant glomerulus in regression (Me) where the obliteration of the capillary and urinary spaces progress; the tissue becomes necrotic. Few segments of the Bowman's capsule persist in areas which are rich in hyaline material (broad arrows) (× 88). (d) Female fetus, 52 days old. The giant glomerulus of the mesonephros (Me) is completely regressed at this stage. Only a few hyalinizing remnants of capsule and excretory tubules (broad arrows) are present. The connecting cord (CC) persists, delimited by a basal lamina and inclused cells with a decreased tinctorial affinity mainly in the intraovarian part (O) (× 40)

next stages, the basal lamina continues to develop gradually in a craniocaudal direction. It first surrounds the whole extragonadal connecting cord and then the intraovarian mass.

Later, in the centre of the ovary of sheep embryo, the germinal and the mesonephric cells form a *compact mass* (day 41) and small cell clusters appear, isolated from this mass. These islets increase their size through a high mitotic activity. They become more numerous and congregate to form regular and branched cords elongated towards the periphery of the ovary. Simultaneously, a connective tissue surrounds these cords and the structures become delimited by a basal lamina which developed at the same time as the elongated cords. Due to the centrifugal direction of the organization process and the gradual evolution, the internal portions of the cords are the most differentiated structures and the external ones the least differentiated[12, 16].

7

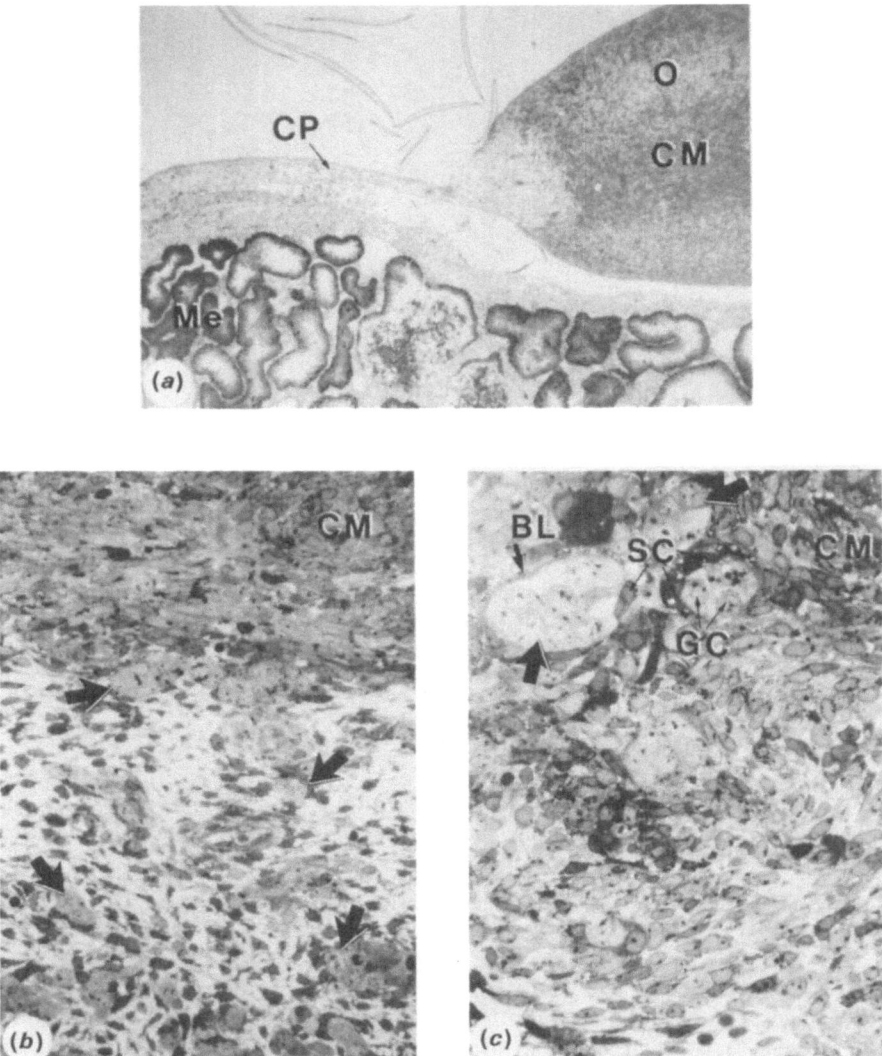

Figure 3 Organization of the ovarian structure. Longitudinal sections of sheep ovary of a 41-day-old fetus, 1 μm thick, stained with toluidine blue. (a) The ovary (O) is always connected with the mesonephros (Me) by the cranial pedunculus (CP), but the connecting cord is invisible on this section. The ovary centre is occupied by a compact mass (CM) of somatic cells originating from the connecting cord. This mass has an irregular aspect due to scattering of mesonephric cells into the surrounding ovarian stroma (× 40). (b) and (c) The clusters (broad arrows) of germinal cells (GC) and somatic cells (SC) become progressively isolated from the compact mass (CM) and extend their development to the ovary surface. A basal lamina (BL) surrounds them to form the ovigerous branch cords showing in section numerous little clusters of germinal and somatic cells not yet surrounded by a basal lamina for those far away from the central mass. The organization of the cords starts from the compact mass (CM) ((b) × 224; (c) × 288)

In the mouse embryo, the ovary of 16 days p.c. is also constructed of a compact mass of mesonephric and germinal cells and the cords are formed with the extensions of the mesonephric tubules. In this case too, the basal lamina develops progressively from the deepest parts of the cords to the most superficial parts[16,17].

Between days 52 and 60 of fetal life in the sheep, the ovary has thus become subdivided into two distinct parts: first, a central mass which is the medulla where the mesonephric cell mass remnants gradually undergo atrophy and hyalinosis and become surrounded by a thick coat of mature, vascular connective tissue; second, a peripheral region, which is the cortex, entirely occupied by radially oriented ovigerous cords which contain a lot of germinal cells in stages of meiotic prophase.

FRAGMENTATION OF THE OVIGEROUS CORDS (Figure 4)

By day 70 of fetal life, the first diplotene stage of the germinal cells appear, as soon as the distal part of the ovigerous cords is separated by connective tissue. The cords contain nests of polyoocytes which arise from degenerative processes in oocytes, and primordial follicles. In the later stages (day 120), the ovigerous cords are substituted almost completely by developing individual follicles surrounded by a basal lamina. So, like any previous developmental and organizational process, follicle formation also appears gradually along a centrifugal direction (from the centre of the ovary to the epithelium surface). The largest and most mature follicles are near the medulla area.

A brief description of the testicular organogenesis demonstrates the same role of the mesonephros (Figure 5). In the embryonic sheep testis from day 29 of fetal life, specific components of the reduced surface stroma under the epithelium differentiate into a tunica albuginea, a structure which does not exist in the ovary. Beginning at the periphery of the testis, the stroma components separate the mesonephric and germinal cell masses. The masses form the seminiferous cords and the testicular and extra-testicular segments of the excretory ducts. The organization of the seminiferous cords progresses in a centripetal direction, opposite to the direction in the ovary. In addition, involution of the giant nephron is limited in the male. The nephron is the site at which the excretory and collecting tubules are transformed into epididymal ducts, and the connecting cord becomes organized into efferent ductules.

So, in the two sexes, the mesonephros *colonizes* the mesenchyme underlying the coelomic epithelium (future germinative epithelium) as soon as the germinal cells reach this area (sheep, day 24 of fetal life[12,16,18]; mouse, day 10.5–11 of fetal life[17]; macaque, day 36–37 of fetal life[18,19]). This view is becoming increasingly accepted. On the other hand, the stages of the gonad development that follow are being interpreted in several divergent ways. The most prudent authors propose a double origin of the somatic cells[13,20].

However, Merchant-Larios and Villalpando[21] have suggested that there is only one origin for the somatic cells in the amphibians. According to a morphological study, they concluded that the cells of the gonadal medulla come from a cellular line arising from the coelomic epithelium and not from the mesonephric blastema. Their hypothesis confirms the interpretation of Humphrey[22]:

after a unilateral sampling of the area containing the mesonephric blastema, he saw the development of the rete cords in the absence of mesonephric tubules.

Results of an experimental mesonephros agenesis of the embryonic chick ovary do not support this hypothesis[23]. This treatment reduces the size of the

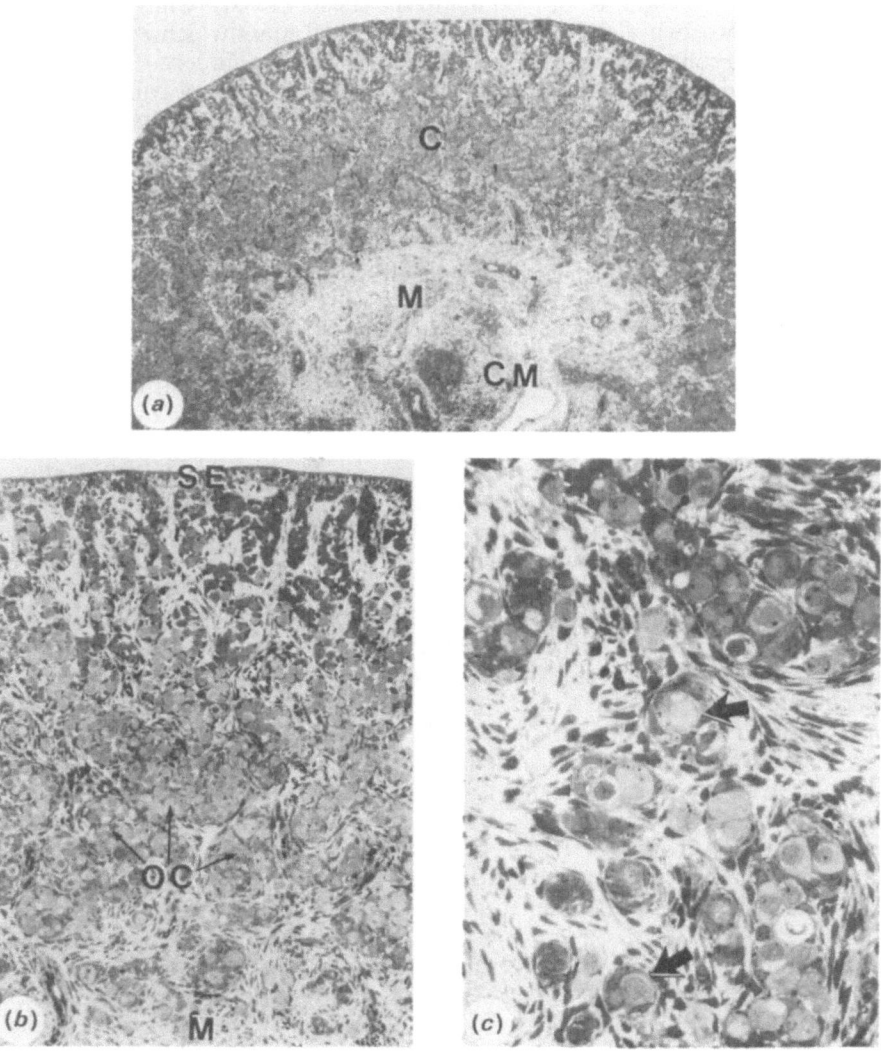

Figure 4 Fragmentation of the ovigerous cords and formation of the primordial follicles. Transverse sections of sheep ovary of a 70-day-old fetus, 1 μm thick, stained with toluidine blue. (a) The remnant of the compact mass (CM) in the medullar ovary centre (M) is surrounded by vascular connective tissue. The cortex (C) is entirely occupied by radially oriented ovigerous cords (× 40). (b) The ovigerous cords (OC) are now well differentiated. They are surrounded with a basal lamina along their entire length; their organization and differentiation has progressed in a centifugal direction from medulla ovary centre (M) to surface epithelium (SE) (× 88). (c) The first follicules (broad arrows) are formed in the more central part of the ovary after the ovigerous cords fragment (× 224)

ovaries, which show typical cell populations (somatic and germinal) but much larger lacunae contained in the medulla and less secondary cords in the cortex and a lack of harmonious development between cortex and medulla. Interpretation of these results is difficult because a histological study confirming the origin of the somatic cells and the relationship between mesonephros and gonad, such as has been done for the mammals, has not been done for the birds.

It has also been proposed that follicular cells of the bird ovaries originate from the germinal epithelium because 'lining bodies' have been found in the granulosa cells[24]. In any case, if organogenesis in birds is different to that in mammals, the somatic cells can also have different origins. Nevertheless, there is little doubt that the mesonephros has an important role in birds, too.

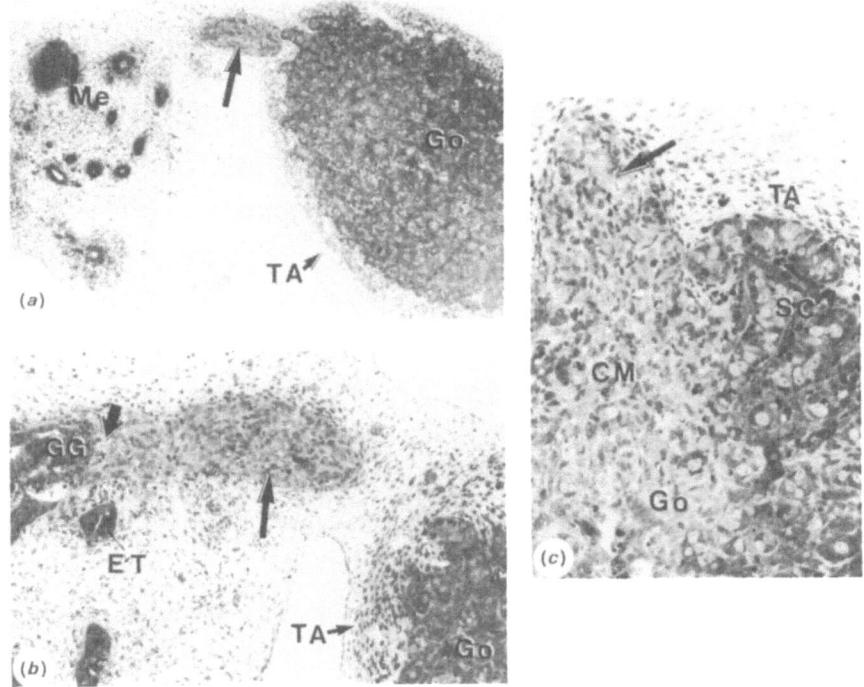

Figure 5 Testicular organogenesis. Longitudinal sections of sheep testis of a 49-day-old fetus, 1 μm thick, stained with toluidine blue.

Similarities with ovarian organogenesis: (1) colonization of the gonad (Go) by mesonephric cells; (2) existence of a connecting cord (thin arrow) between the mesonephros (Me) and the gonad (Go); (3) giant glomerulus involution of the mesonephros (Me) with hyalinizing deposit formation at the Bowman's capsule often missing (broad arrow).

Differences with ovarian morphogenesis: (1) formation of an external tunica albuginea (TA); (2) organization of the seminiferous cords (SC) which progress in a centripetal direction in contrast to the centrifugal in ovigerous cords; (3) giant glomerulus (GG) does not undergo regression as do the others in the caudal region of the mesonephros but becomes the site of the entire system of testicular cords and excurrent ducts.

In the male, there is an anatomic continuity between the seminiferous cords (SC) in the testis and excretory and collecting tubules (ET) of the giant nephron (Me) via the connecting cord (thin arrow) and the central mass (CM) which become organized into ductuli efferentes. ((a) × 32; (b) × 71; (c) × 117)

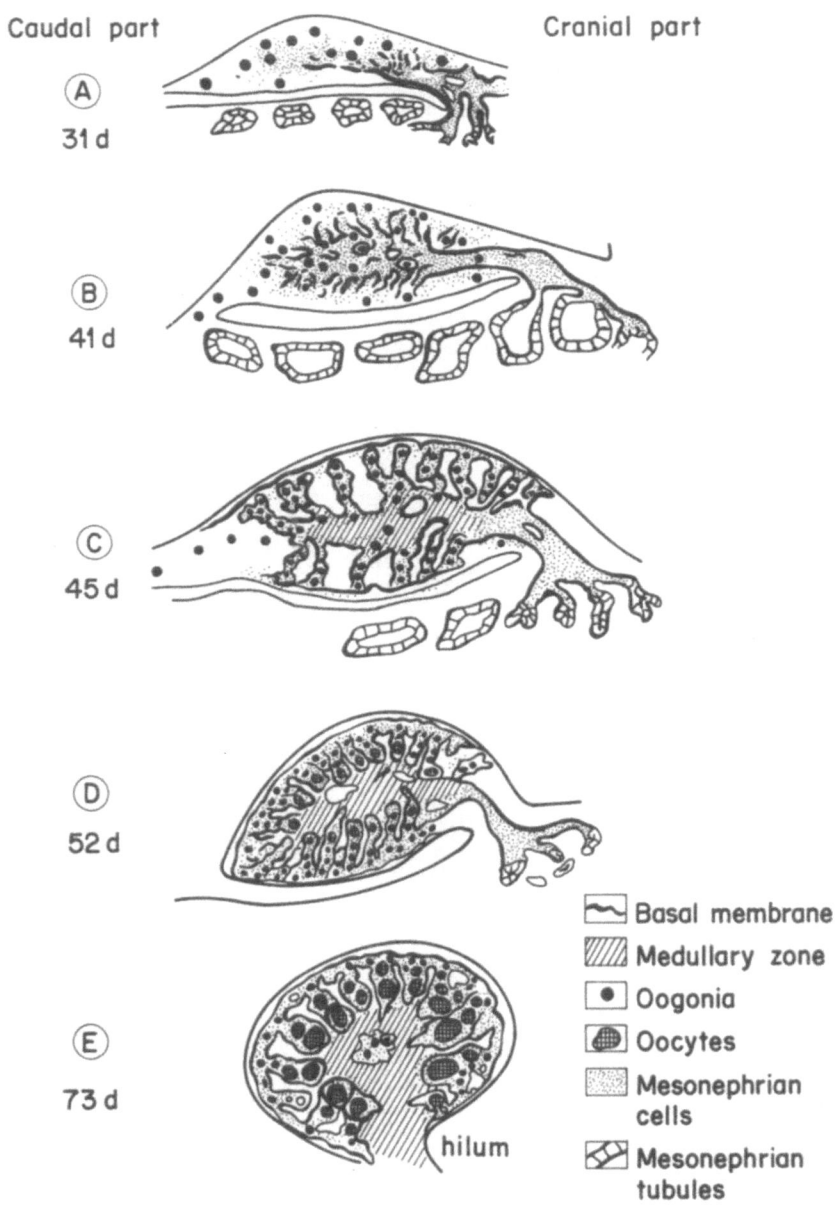

Figure 6 Schematic representation of sheep ovary organogenesis. d = Days. (A) Colonization of the gonad (longitudinal section: × 30). (B–D) Connecting cord between mesonephros and gonad. Organization of the ovigerous cords from the central mass (longitudinal section: (B) × 30; (C) × 30; (D) × 18). (E) Fragmentation of the ovigerous cords. Formation of the primordial follicles (transverse section: × 18)

In mammals, interaction between germinal cells and somatic cells contributes to the development of the ovary. Indeed, destruction of the primordial germ cells of the rat (with the cytotoxic action of busulfan) does not prevent the sexual differentiation[25]. On the contrary, the somatic cells of the sex cords, in the absence of oocytes, are unable to form follicles[26]. Likewisè, no cÿtodifferentiation of steroidogenic cells takes place in the ovary without germ cells which prevent the formation of follicles during the post-natal development. Steroidogenic tissue is only formed in the presence of a small number of follicles which become atretic[27].

So, the morphogenesis of the ovary depends on an interaction between germinal cells and somatic cells which influences the processes of follicular development and atresia and establishes the interstitial gland[28].

Even if contradictory hypotheses do exist due to insufficient experimental demonstrations and to subjective interpretations from the same morphological facts, the involvement of the mesonephros in gonadal morphogenesis is a major developmental mechanism in mammalian embryology. We have summarized our ideas in a schematic representation based on the ovarian organogenesis in sheep embryo (Figure 6).

Acknowledgements

This chapter summarizes results published in collaboration with Dr L. Zamboni[12, 16, 18]. The two authors of this review have added only some new ideas and discussion.

We would like to thank Mr Martin Graeme for his translation.

References

1. Carlon, N. and Stahl, A. (1973). Les premiers stades du développement des gonades chez l'homme et les vertébrés supérieurs. *Path. Biol.,* **21**, 903–14
2. Mauleon, P. and Mariana, J. C. (1977). Oogenesis and folliculogenesis. In Cole, H. H. and Cupps, P. T., (eds.) *Reproduction in Domestic Animals,* 3rd edn., pp. 175–202. (London: Academic Press)
3. Waldeyer, W. (1870). *Eierstock und Ei.* (Leipzig: Englemann)
4. Balfour (1878). On the structure and development of vertebrate ovary. *Q. J. Microsc. Sci.,* **18**, 1–81
5. Coert, H. J. (1898). *Over de outwikkeling en den bouw van de geschlachtsklier bix de zoogdieren, meer en het bejzonder van den eierstok.* Thesis, Proefschrift, Leiden
6. Witschi, E. (1951). Embryogenesis of the adrenal and the reproductive glands. In Pincus, G. (ed.) *Recent Progress in Hormone Research,* Vol. 6, pp. 1–27. (New York: Academic Press)
7. Jost, A. (1972). Données préliminaires sur les stades initiaux de la différenciation du testicule chez le rat. *Arch. Anat. Microsc. Morphol. Exp.,* **61**, 415–38
8. Byskov, A. G. and Lintern-Moore, S. (1973). Follicle formation in the immature mouse ovary: the role of the rete ovarii. *J. Anat.,* **116**, 207–17
9. Byskov, A. G. (1975). The role of the rete ovarii in meiosis and follicle formation in different mammalian species. *J. Reprod. Fertil.,* **45**, 201–9
10. Deanesly, R. (1975). Follicle formation in guinea pigs and rabbits: A comparative study with notes on the rete ovarii. *J. Reprod. Fertil.,* **45**, 371–4
11. Witschi, E. (1956). *Development of Vertebrates,* pp. 154–7. (Philadelphia: Saunders)
12. Zamboni, L., Bezard, J. and Mauleon, P. (1979). The role of the mesonephros in the development of the sheep fetal ovary. *Ann. Biol. Anim. Bioch. Biophys.,* **19**, 1153–78
·13. Fouquet, J. P. and Dang, D. C. (1980). A comparative study of the development of the fetal testis and ovary in the monkey (*Macaca fascicularis*). *Reprod. Nutr. Dev.,* **20**, 1439–59
14. Zuckerman, S. and Baker, T. G. (1977). The development of the ovary and the process of oogenesis. In Zuckerman, S. and Weir, B. J. (eds.) *The Ovary,* Vol. 1, 2nd edn., pp. 42–68. (New York: Academic Press)
15. Brenñer, J. L. (1915). The mesonephric corpuscle of the sheep, cow and deer. *Anat. Rec.,* **10**, 1–6

16. Zamboni, L., Upadhyay, S., Bezard, J. and Mauleon, P. (1980). The role of the mesonephros in the development of the mammalian ovary. In Tozzini, R. I., Reeves, G. and Pineda, R. L. (eds.) *Endocrine Physiopathology of the Ovary*, pp. 4–42. (Amsterdam: Elsevier, North Holland Biomedical Press)

17. Upadhyay, S., Luciani, J. M. and Zamboni, L. (1979). The role of the mesonephros in the development of indifferent gonads and ovaries of the mouse. *Ann. Biol. Anim. Bioch. Biophys.*, **19**, 1179–96

18. Zamboni, L., Upadhyay, S., Bezard, J. and Mauleon, P. (1981). The role of the mesonephros in the development of the sheep testis and its excurrent pathways. In Byskov, A. G. and Peters, H. (eds.) *Development and Function of Reproductive Organs*, pp. 31–40. (Amsterdam: Excerpta Medica)

19. Dang, D. C. and Fouquet, J. P. (1979). Differentiation of the fetal gonad of *Macaca fascicularis* with special reference to the testis. *Ann. Biol. Anim. Bioch. Biophys.*, **19**, 1197–1210

20. Merchant-Larios, H. (1978). Ovarian differentiation. In Jones, E. (ed.) *The Vertebrate Ovary*, pp. 47–81. (New York: Plenum Press)

21. Merchant-Larios, H. and Villapando, I. (1981). Ultrastructural events during early gonadal development in *Rana pipiens* and *Xenopus laevis*. *Anat. Rec.*, **199**, 349–60

22. Humphrey, R. R. (1933). The development and sex differentiation of the gonad in the wood frog (*Rana sylvatica*) following extirpation or orthotopic implantation of the intermediate segment and adjacent mesoderm. *J. Exp. Zool.*, **65**, 243–69

23. Popova, L. and Scheib, D. (1981). Différenciation ovarienne chez l'embryon de Poulet après agénésie expérimentale du mésonéphros. *Arch. Anat. Micr. Morphol. Exp.*, **70**, 189–204

24. Bellairs, R. (1965). The relationship between oocyte and follicle in the hen's ovary as shown by electron microscopy. *J. Embryol. Exp. Morphol.*, **13**, 215–33

25. Merchant, H. (1975). Rat gonadal and ovarian organogenesis with and without germ cells. An ultrastructural study. *Dev. Biol.*, **44**, 1–21

26. Merchant-Larios, H. (1979). Follicular atresia and the formation of an interstitial gland. *Eur. J. Obstet. Gynaecol. Reprod. Biol.*, **9**, 219

27. Merchant-Larios, H. (1976). The role of germ cells in the morphogenesis and cytodifferentiation of the rat ovary. In Müller-Bérat, N. (ed.) *Progress in Differentiation Research*, pp. 453–62. (Amsterdam: North-Holland)

28. Merchant-Larios, H. and Centeno, B. (1981). Morphogenesis of the ovary from the sterile W/Wv mouse. In *Advances in the Morphology of Cells and Tissues*, pp. 383–92. (New York: A. R. Liss)

II—Ovarian Follicle Biodynamics

2
Hormonal control of ovarian follicular development

J. S. Richards

INTRODUCTION

In adult female mammals follicular growth is initiated continuously irrespective of physiological status, including pregnancy, lactation or other interruptions of cyclicity[1]. Although the stimulus for growth is not yet known, early development of the follicle comprises enlargement of the oocyte, proliferation of surrounding granulosa cells and the organization of a definitive theca cell layer external to the basement membrane. Continuous growth of follicles from the preantral stage through antrum formation and the time of ovulation is dependent largely on the pituitary hormones, follicle-stimulating hormone (FSH) and luteinizing hormone (LH). The entire process of growth and cell differentiation of any given follicle appears to comprise progressive changes in the response of follicular (theca and granulosa) cells to the two pituitary gonadotrophins[2].

The change in response of follicular cells to the gonadotrophins is dependent, in turn, on the ability of follicles to produce the steroid hormone, oestradiol. Oestradiol acts synergistically with the gonadotrophins to alter follicular cell differentiation. Thus, only developing preovulatory follicles produce oestradiol and only those follicles producing oestradiol develop the mechanisms necessary to respond to the LH surge, ovulate and luteinize (Figure 1).

KINETICS OF FOLLICULAR GROWTH

The schematic diagram of follicular growth as illustrated in Figure 2 has been derived primarily from the kinetic analyses of follicular growth in the mouse[3,4] and hamster[5], but also from an analytical model of ovarian follicular dynamics[6] and a morphological analysis of follicular development in the rat[7]. The upper panel illustrates the pattern of serum concentrations of gonadotrophins FSH and LH in the 4–5 day oestrous cycle[8–10] and during pregnancy[11]. A surge of both FSH and LH occurs late in the afternoon of proestrus while the FSH surge extends into the morning of oestrus. If pregnancy occurs serum concentrations of the gonadotrophins remain low until the last 4 days preceding parturition.

17

As serum progesterone declines between days 19 and 23 of pregnancy, there is a subtle, sustained increase in basal LH[11,12].

The lower portion of Figure 2 depicts the relative changes in follicle size, from small preantral follicles possessing one or two layers of granulosa cells to large antral follicles that have greater than four layers of granulosa cells and are characterized by a large fluid-filled cavity (antrum) in which the oocyte is suspended. Time in days is plotted on the x-axis. Graafian follicles ovulating in response to the gonadotrophin surge of one cycle, as indicated, begin to grow at least 19 days earlier as part of a larger pool of growing follicles. Thus, once committed to grow, a follicle is exposed to three or more consecutive surges of gonadotrophins (if pregnancy does not occur) or to elevated serum concentrations of progesterone (if pregnancy does occur). In the adult rat most of these follicles grow continuously until, as small antral follicles, they undergo atresia. Only a few follicles enter the final stages of maturation. It has been proposed that the surge of gonadotrophins in the cycle preceding ovulation selects from the pool of preantral or small antral follicles those that will ovulate and luteinize at the next proestrus[7,13,14]. However, this argument does not explain the development of preovulatory follicles which occurs during days 19–23 of pregnancy. At this time follicular growth is dependent on the subtle, sustained rise in serum concentrations of LH, not FSH, which occurs as serum concentrations of progesterone decline[12,15].

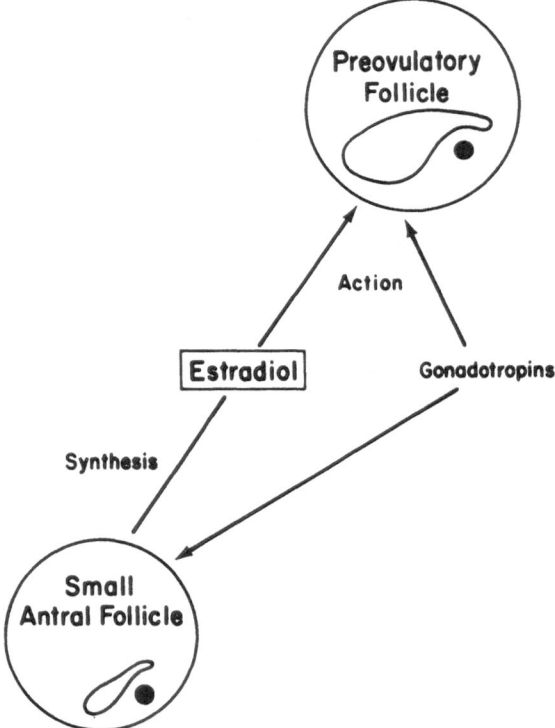

Figure 1 The development of preovulatory follicles is dependent on increased synthesis of oestradiol and the synergistic actions of oestradiol and the gonadotrophins on granulosa cell differentiation

From the scheme depicted in Figure 2, it would be predicted that a large number of follicles arrive at the small antral stage of growth each day. Those reaching this stage when progesterone is elevated and serum LH is low degenerate. Only those small antral follicles which appear on days 19–20 of pregnancy become exposed to the rising concentrations of LH, continue to develop, and eventually ovulate. Reasons for the importance of LH as well as FSH in the development of preovulatory follicles will be discussed in the following sections.

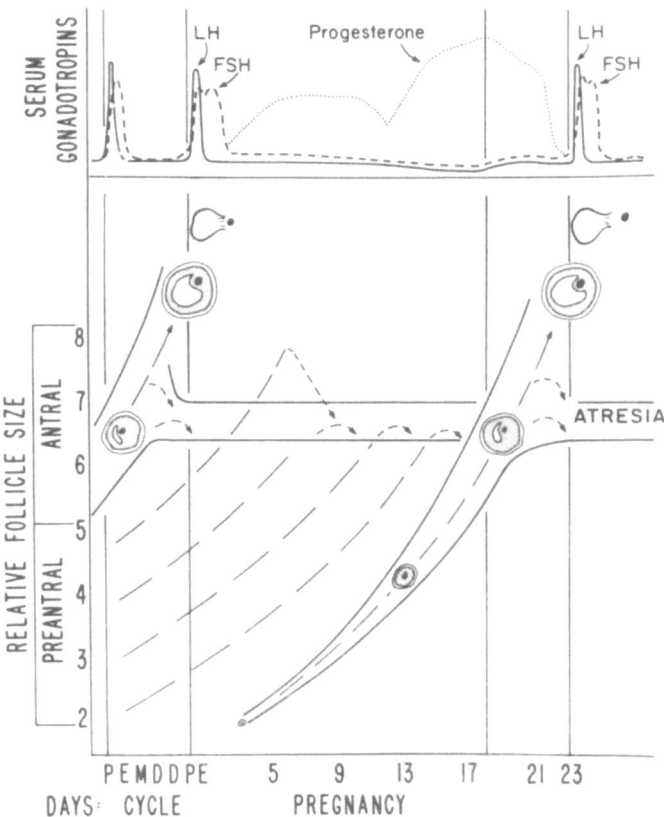

Figure 2 Schematic diagram of follicular growth in the pregnant rat (see text)

RECEPTORS FOR FSH IN FOLLICULAR DEVELOPMENT

FSH, as suggested by its name, has been shown to have a primary role in maintaining ovarian follicular development[16,17]. Autoradiographic and binding analyses have revealed that receptors for FSH are localized exclusively in granulosa cells (Figure 3)[18,19]. Further, granulosa cells of follicles at all stages of development appear to possess receptors for FSH suggesting that these binding sites are a constitutive component of the granulosa cell plasma membrane. This idea is supported by evidence that FSH binding sites are retained in granulosa cells of hypophysectomized rats[19] and that even after hypophysectomy, FSH can stimulate in granulosa cells cAMP accumulation[20], proliferation[21], increased intracellular cAMP binding sites[22] and increased FSH receptor content[19,23].

From the preceding observations, it seems that FSH acts to enhance its own FSH receptor-cAMP response system in granulosa cells of follicles at all stages of growth until ovulation. This is emphasized further by the apparent reversibility of FSH responsiveness in granulosa cells of preantral follicles exposed to elevated amounts of FSH. For example, when sufficient FSH is administered *in vivo* to cause rapid desensitization of granulosa cell cAMP accumulation, the refractory phase is transient[24]. Within 12–24 h after the onset of desensitization, FSH stimulation of cAMP accumulation is clearly demonstrable once again. Further, FSH appears unable to induce a loss of FSH receptor during follicular growth even in response to doses of hormone which desensitize cAMP accumulation[24]. The reversibility of desensitization to FSH observed in preantral follicles contrasts with the irreversible effects that occur during luteinization when both FSH responsive cAMP accumulation[25] and FSH binding sites are lost[19,26].

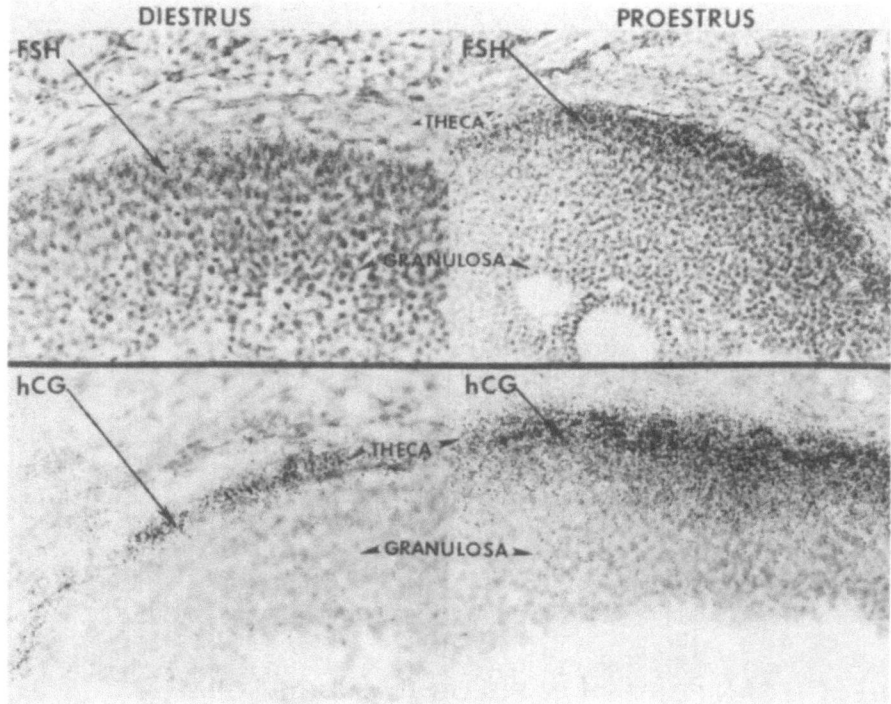

Figure 3 Localization of [125I]hFSH and [125I]hCG in antral follicles of adult dioestrous and proestrous rats. 125I-labelled hormones were injected intravenously. After 2 h the rats were killed and the ovaries were excised, fixed in Bouin's solution, embedded and sectioned. The sections were prepared for autoradiography and subsequently developed. Note the specific localization of [125I]hFSH on granulosa cells of follicles present on dioestrus and proestrus. In contrast, [125I]hCG is bound to theca cells of follicles present on dioestrus and proestrus but is only bound to granulosa cells of proestrous follicles

If responsiveness to FSH, therefore, is maintained, even ensured and enhanced by FSH, throughout follicular growth, why do so many follicles degenerate and become atretic? At this juncture one has to consider other events which act to alter the response of granulosa cells, not only to FSH but also to LH.

LH AND RECEPTORS FOR LH DURING FOLLICULAR GROWTH

Luteinizing hormone, as the name suggests, has a primary role in stimulating ovulation and luteinization. In addition to the LH surge, however, it is poignantly clear that small but sustained increases in basal concentrations of LH, but not FSH, play an essential and critical role in determining which follicles enter the final stages of preovulatory growth[12, 15, 17, 27–30].

Autoradiographic and binding analyses have revealed that receptors for LH are localized and may be constitutive membrane components of theca cells but appear on membranes of granulosa cells only in developing preovulatory follicles (Figure 3)[19, 31–33]. These observations suggest that although LH may act only on theca cells of small follicles the hormone acts on both theca and granulosa cells of large follicles *prior* to ovulation. The role of LH in follicular cell function *prior* to the LH surge is obligatory for preovulatory follicular growth. This will be illustrated by describing the changes in follicular cell function in the pregnant rat in which ovulation occurs immediately postpartum. Although not yet conclusively demonstrated in the rat, similar changes in LH are presumed to occur during the oestrous cycle and at puberty.

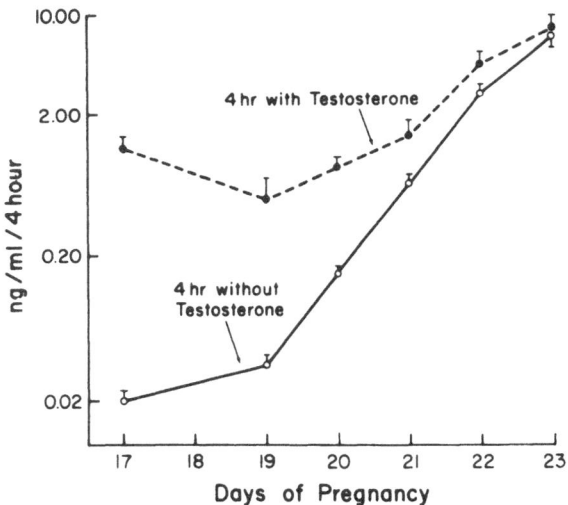

Figure 4 Oestradiol accumulation by follicles *in vitro*. Follicles were isolated from ovaries of rats on days 17–23 of pregnancy. Follicles were incubated individually in 500 μl medium 199 containing 10 mmol l^{-1} HEPES with or without exogenous testosterone. All incubations were run for 4 h at 37°C under 95% O_2 : 5% CO_2. Oestradiol accumulated in the presence of testosterone reflects total follicular (granulosa cell) aromatase activity. Oestradiol accumulated in the absence of substrate reflects the ability of follicles (theca) to produce androgen substrate. Note that between days 19 and 23 both endogenous androgen synthesis as well as aromatase activity increase markedly. Data are expressed on a logarithmic scale

Pregnant rat

From days 2–19 of pregnancy in the rat, follicles continuously reach the small antral stage of development (Figure 2). In the absence of appropriate stimulation, these follicles are destined to become atretic and never gain the functional competence of preovulatory follicles. Granulosa cells of these small antral follicles are similar to those isolated on dioestrus of the oestrous cycle[32]. They possess abundant receptor for FSH as well as an active aromatase enzyme system capable of converting exogenous testosterone to oestradiol (Figure 4)[15,32]. Therefore, it is not a lack of either serum FSH or granulosa cell FSH receptor content that ultimately leads to atresia. Rather, atresia appears to occur as a consequence of low serum LH, minimal theca cell androgen synthesis, and low LH receptor concentrations in both theca and granulosa cells[12,15].

Although granulosa cells of small antral follicles have aromatase activity, whole follicles incubated *in vitro* without exogenous androgen substrate fail to accumulate oestradiol (Figure 4)[15]. Since theca cells have been shown to be the follicular site of androgen production[29,34], we have postulated that serum concentrations of LH determine the production of theca cell androgens in small follicles and thereby *also* determine follicular oestradiol production (Figure 4). Oestradiol, in turn, is required to enhance FSH induction of LH receptors in granulosa cells[2,19]. Acquisition of LH receptors in granulosa cells, in conjunction with other oestradiol–FSH induced functions, now permits granulosa cells to differentiate in response to progressive increases in LH until the LH surge initiates ovulation and luteinization. Evidence to support the hypothesis illustrated in Figure 5 and outlined above has been derived from several experiments discussed below.

Neutralization of LH

At the end of pregnancy (days 19–23) in the rat, serum progesterone declines and basal concentrations of serum LH increase[11,12]. In association with increased

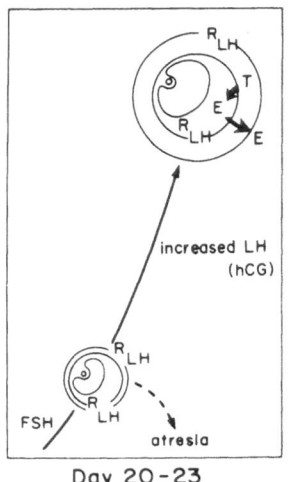

Day 20-23

I. FSH supports the growth of small antral follicles during pregnancy.

II. Increased LH/hCG is required for the final growth and differentiation of preovulatory follicles.

III. LH/hCG increases:

Theca	Granulosa
LH Receptor	LH Receptor
↓	↓
Androgen Synthesis	Aromatase Activity

IV. The action of LH/hCG on aromatase activity appears to be mediated by cAMP.

Figure 5 Schematic diagram of functional changes in theca and granulosa cells of developing preovulatory follicles

serum LH, progressive increases in LH receptor content in both granulosa cells and theca cells occur. These progressive increases in LH receptor can be blocked by the administration of an LH specific antiserum[15].

The elevations in serum LH and follicular cell LH receptor content are associated with marked, progressive increases in the ability of individual follicles to accumulate oestradiol when incubated *in vitro* without exogenous androgen substrate (Figure 4)[15]. As stated previously, aromatase activity (oestradiol accumulation by follicles incubated with testosterone substrate) is present in the small antral follicles isolated on all days of pregnancy. However, aromatase activity also increases between days 19 and 23 of pregnancy (Figure 4) and this five-fold increase can be blocked by LH antiserum. Taken together these results indicate that follicular oestradiol accumulation *in vitro* is dependent on the ability of theca cells to produce aromatizable androgen substrates. Theca androgen production, in turn, appears critically dependent on subtle, sustained increases in LH, not FSH[29].

Effects of exogenous human chorionic gonadotrophin

As indicated in Figure 2, serum concentrations of LH are low between days 14 and 16 of pregnancy. The antral follicles present at this time are small, contain low LH receptor content, produce little or no oestradiol, and do not ovulate in response to a bolus of 20 IU hCG[15]. To examine the effects of small, sustained increases in LH activity on these follicles, low and increasing concentrations (0.25–1.5 IU) of hCG were administered to pregnant rats on days 14–15. These low amounts of hCG, given twice daily for 2 days, stimulated the growth of follicles and increased LH receptor content in granulosa cells in a time- and dose-dependent manner[12]. These increases in LH receptor were associated with progressive increases in follicular oestradiol accumulation reaching 500-fold in response to the *in vivo* administration of 1.5 IU hCG. These follicles were functionally indistinguishable from preovulatory follicles present on day 23 of pregnancy (Figure 4) and would ovulate in response to a bolus injection of 20 IU hCG[12]. The increase in follicular oestradiol production in response to the low amounts of hCG can be attributed primarily to a marked increase in endogenous androgen production[29]. These results support the hypothesis that although FSH can maintain the growth of a certain number of small antral follicles, an increase in serum LH is required to stimulate follicular oestradiol production and the development of preovulatory follicles (Figure 5). Furthermore, the results of these studies suggest that even in the presence of elevated serum progesterone, subtle increases in serum LH can stimulate follicular growth. Thus, the inhibitory effects of progesterone on follicular growth appear to be mediated primarily by negative feedback suppression of LH secretion rather than by a direct inhibitory action on follicular cell function.

OESTRADIOL AND FSH IN FOLLICULAR CELL FUNCTION

By the 1940s it was well established that oestradiol but not testosterone would increase ovarian responsiveness to gonadotrophins *in vivo*[35, 36]. In the 1960s a direct action of oestradiol and the localization of oestradiol binding in the ovary were first demonstrated[37, 38]. By the 1970s the specific intraovarian localization of FSH receptors in granulosa cells was revealed by autoradiography[18]. At this time Goldenberg *et al.*[39] re-examined the role of oestrogens and demonstrated that prolonged treatment of hypophysectomized rats with the non-steroidal oestrogen diethylstilboestrol increased ovarian uptake of [^{3}H]FSH *in vivo*. Identification and quantitation of oestradiol binding to granulosa cell nuclei have provided further evidence that granulosa cells are an intraovarian target tissue for oestradiol[40]. Collectively, these observations provoked new interest and prompted two questions. (1) Was the oestrogen-induced increase in ovarian uptake of [^{3}H]FSH *in vivo* related to an increased number of granulosa cells per ovary or to an increased number of FSH receptors per granulosa cell? (2) Was increased ovarian responsiveness to gonadotrophins related to the number of FSH receptors? The studies described below indicate that (1) oestradiol alone does not increase the number of FSH receptors per granulosa cell; and (2) therefore oestradiol-mediated enhancement of follicular responsiveness to FSH is not dependent on a change in FSH receptor content in granulosa cells.

The interactions of oestradiol and FSH on granulosa cell function have been examined primarily in hypophysectomized immature rats treated sequentially with oestradiol followed by highly purified hFSH. These treatments stimulate the sequential development of large preantral and then antral follicles[19, 40].

When the effects of these hormones on granulosa cell proliferation were examined, oestradiol was found to increase the proliferation of granulosa cells[21, 39]. This was observed when proliferation was measured either as DNA content of isolated cells or as per cent of labelled cells observed after *in vivo* administration of [^{3}H]thymidine and subsequent autoradiographic analyses[21]. However, even in the presence of oestradiol, granulosa cell proliferation was not sustained as indicated by the decrease in the labelling index and by the plateau in granulosa cell DNA content. If, however, FSH was given to the oestradiol-treated rats, a new burst of proliferative activity followed. This proliferative phase was also not sustained[21]. Thus, each hormone exhibited a specific but limited capacity to evoke a proliferative response in granulosa cells. These results have suggested that a steroid hormone (oestradiol) and a protein hormone (FSH), each presumably acting via different intracellular mechanisms, have limited capacities to promote granulosa cell proliferation[41]. Whether or not these hormones directly stimulate granulosa cell proliferation is an area which is not completely resolved because factors present in serum have recently been shown to stimulate marked proliferation of granulosa cells in culture[42]. Therefore, a synergistic effect of these hormones and serum factors may be involved. Nevertheless, stimulation by specific hormones at distinct developmental stages seems to be required for the apparent continuous nature of follicular growth.

The synergistic effects of oestradiol and FSH on granulosa cell receptors for gonadotrophins are summarized in Figure 6. Oestradiol alone had no effect on the number of FSH or LH receptors per granulosa cell[19, 43]. Thus, the increased ovarian uptake of [^{3}H]FSH *in vivo* after prolonged oestrogen treatment[39] reflects the increased number of granulosa cells per ovary and not an increase in the number of FSH receptors per granulosa cell. Since the oestradiol-induced responsiveness of granulosa cells to FSH is increased, but not related to changes in FSH receptor number, the question of how oestradiol enhances FSH stimulation of granulosa cell differentiation and the appearance of LH receptor remains.

Some possible mechanisms by which oestradiol might act to enhance the responsiveness of granulosa cells to FSH are summarized below. Nuclear

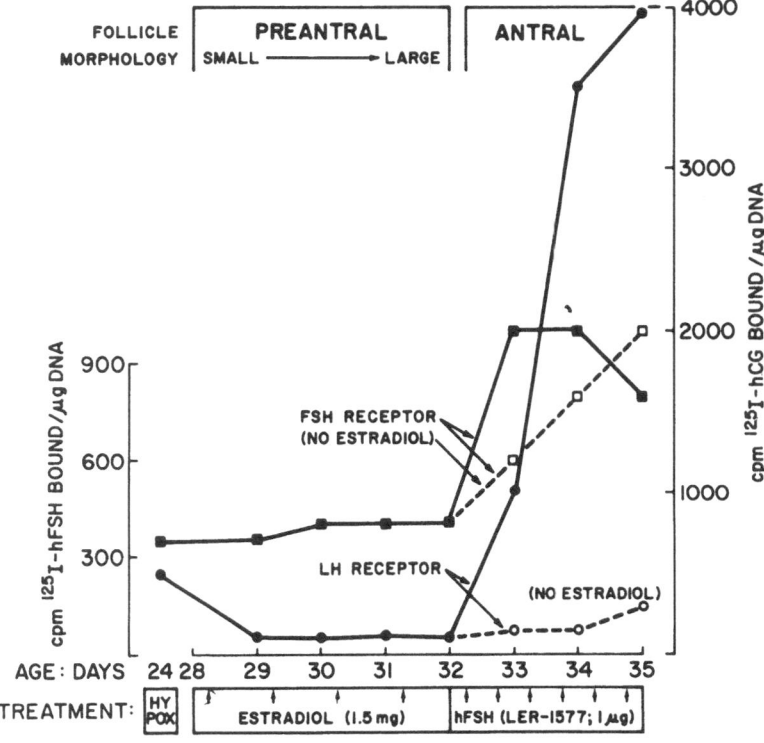

Figure 6 Changes in receptors for FSH and LH in granulosa cells of preantral and antral follicles of hormonally primed hypophysectomized immature rats. FSH receptor is unchanged by treatment of hypophysectomized rats with oestradiol. However, FSH alone increases the content of receptors for FSH, and oestradiol enhances the rate of this increase. In contrast, receptors for LH/hCG in granulosa cells are not induced by FSH alone. Only if rats are pretreated with oestradiol does LH receptor appear on granulosa cells (From references 19 and 23.)

receptors for oestradiol have been preferentially localized in nuclei of isolated granulosa cells, as distinguished from residual ovarian tissue remaining after isolation of granulosa cells[40]. Furthermore, nuclear oestradiol–receptor content was high during follicular development and low in association with atresia and early luteinization[40]. Thus, it seems reasonable to propose that the effects of oestradiol on granulosa cell function are mediated in a fashion similar to that reported for other target tissues, i.e. via the translocation of the cytosol oestradiol–receptor complex to the nucleus. Binding of the oestradiol–receptor complex to nuclear 'acceptor' sites presumably results in altered genomic expression, the synthesis of new messenger RNA, and a change in any one of a number of the component parts of the FSH receptor response system in granulosa cells. For example, oestradiol could act to modify the number of FSH receptors. As already discussed, however, oestradiol acts elsewhere. Since FSH has been shown to stimulate production of cAMP[24, 25, 44], and since cAMP has been implicated as a second messenger of protein hormone action[45], including now the induction of LH receptor[46], it is possible that oestradiol enhances the ability of FSH to stimulate cAMP production. Alternatively, oestradiol might increase intracellular concentrations of cAMP dependent protein kinases. Or oestradiol may increase the synthesis of a protein which is the substrate for cAMP dependent phosphorylation. Although these alternatives are by no means exhaustive, they have provided a framework to discuss studies which have been done to determine the mechanism by which oestradiol increases the responsiveness of ovarian granulosa cells to FSH[27].

The ability of oestradiol to enhance FSH stimulation of cAMP production in intact granulosa cells as well as in membrane preparations has been examined. Both *in vivo* and *in vitro* studies indicate that granulosa cells of oestradiol-treated rats exhibit a two-fold greater stimulation of cAMP in response to FSH than do cells of hypophysectomized rats[20, 47]. Furthermore, the amounts of FSH required to stimulate a demonstrable dose-dependent increase in cAMP concentrations in

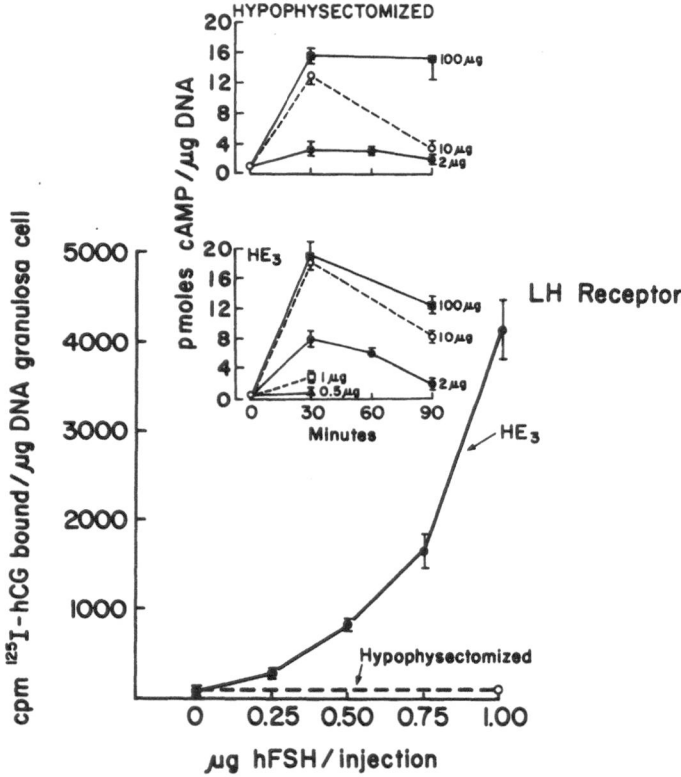

Figure 7 Dose-dependent increases in cAMP and receptor for LH in granulosa cells of hypophysectomized (H) rats treated with or without oestradiol (E) for 3 days. Hypophysectomized rats or hypophysectomized rats treated with oestradiol (HE$_3$) were injected twice daily for 2 days with increasing doses (0.25–1.0 µg) of highly purified hFSH (LER—117/8). Only rats treated with oestradiol exhibited a dose-dependent increase in LH receptor. To examine the ability of these same doses of hormone to stimulate cAMP accumulation, H rats and HE$_3$ rats were given similar doses of hFSH intravenously. At 30, 60 and 90 min rats were killed, granulosa cells were rapidly expressed from the ovaries placed in boiling water for 5 min. cAMP was measured by radioimmunoassay. Note that although granulosa cells of H rats produce cAMP in response to hFSH, LH receptor is not induced. Note also that the amounts of cAMP accumulated in granulosa cells of HE$_3$ rats is approximately two-fold higher than that produced by cells of H rats (From reference 19.)

granulosa cells *in vivo* correspond to the doses of hormone required to induce LH receptors in granulosa cells *in vivo* (Figure 7)[20]. This enhancement by oestradiol of FSH stimulation of cAMP accumulation and adenylate cyclase activity[47] occurs without a change in the number of receptors for FSH. Thus, some component of the FSH-responsive adenylate cyclase system appears to be modified. Even greater increases in FSH-responsive adenylate cyclase activity are observed when hypophysectomized rats are treated with both oestradiol and FSH suggesting that components of the cyclase system itself are also regulated by the synergistic effects of the steroid and the gonadotrophin (Figure 8)[47]. Similarly, proestrous follicles of adult cycling rats[25, 32] and pregnant rats[15] exhibit a marked increase in FSH-responsive adenylate cyclase and cAMP accumulation without changes in the number of receptors for FSH. Presumably it is the rising concentrations of follicular oestradiol which are responsible for the enhancement of gonadotrophin responsive adenylate cyclase (Figure 5).

Intracellular concentrations of cAMP specific binding sites and cAMP dependent protein kinase activity have also been examined[22]. The results reveal that oestradiol alone had no effect on the number of cAMP binding sites in granulosa

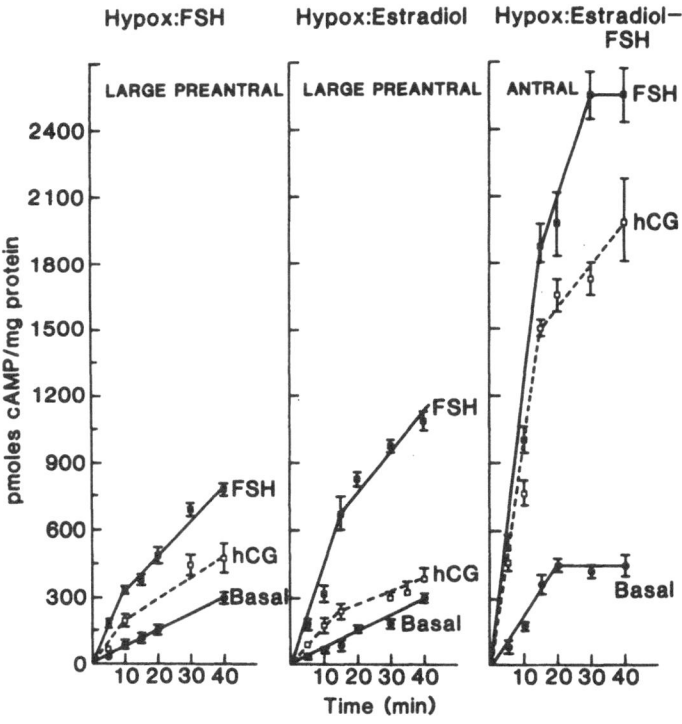

Figure 8 Hormone response adenylate cyclase activity in hypophysectomized (Hypox) rats treated with FSH for 3 days, oestradiol for 3 days or oestradiol followed by FSH. Note the two-fold increase in FSH-responsive cyclase after oestradiol treatment and the synergistic effect of oestradiol and FSH. Note also that receptors for FSH in rats treated with FSH alone or with oestradiol followed by FSH are the same (Figure 6). Thus, the increase in FSH-responsive cyclase as well as LH-responsive cyclase includes a change in some component of the cyclase system other than the receptor (From reference 47.)

cell cytosol preparations but the steroid did enhance the ability of FSH to increase cAMP binding 10–20-fold. This effect is reminiscent of the oestradiol-mediated enhancement of FSH induction of LH receptor (Figure 6) and adenylate cyclase activity (Figure 8)[47]. The biological function of the cAMP binding protein has been shown to be the regulatory subunit of type II cAMP dependent protein kinase[22]. These data indicate that FSH, and therefore presumably cAMP, is regulating the intracellular concentrations of its own cAMP dependent protein kinase. Thus, FSH and cAMP appear to exert positive effects on their own response systems in differentiating granulosa cells.

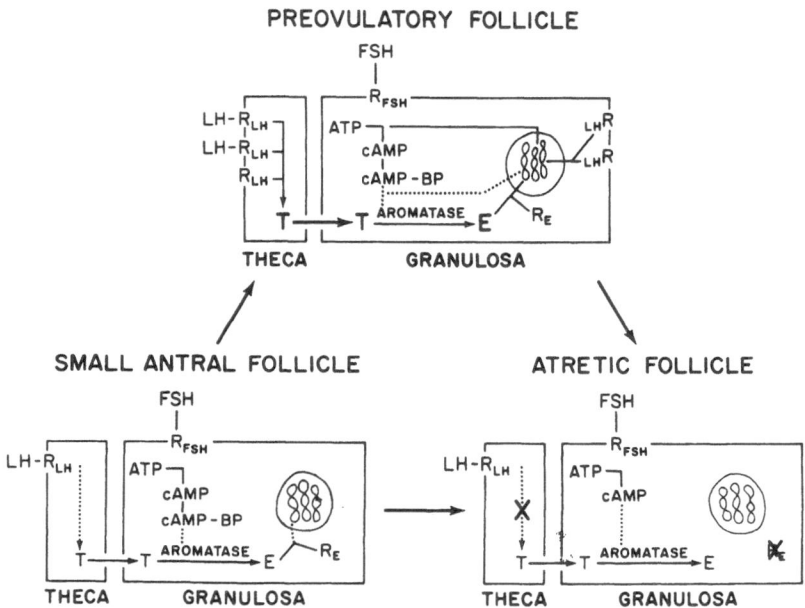

Figure 9 Summary of preovulatory follicular growth in the intact adult rat during oestrous cycle or at the end of pregnancy

The interactions of oestradiol, FSH and LH are summarized schematically in Figure 9. At least during the oestrous cycle and at the end of pregnancy in the rat, the growth of preovulatory follicles seems to require increased synthesis of oestradiol. This appears to depend on increased responsiveness of theca cells to subtle increases in serum LH and subsequent increased production of thecal-derived androgens. Thus, the theca cell may hold the clue to what conditions permit preovulatory follicular growth. Follicles in which theca cells do not develop responsiveness to LH and which do not produce androgens or oestradiol may become atretic.

In addition, preovulatory follicular growth is dependent on the interactions of oestradiol, FSH and LH. As discussed above, the FSH–cAMP response system in small antral follicles present on dioestrus or in the middle of pregnancy appears adequate to maintain some aromatase activity in granulosa cells. With increased production of thecal androgen, oestradiol production also increases and then oestradiol assumes the director's role in determining subsequent granulosa cell differentiation: induction of LH receptor, increased amounts of adenylate cyclase, increased concentrations of cAMP dependent protein kinase and increased aromatase activity. These as well as other events provide the follicles with the mechanisms to respond to the LH surge, ovulate and luteinize. Without these final developmental changes it appears that oocytes would remain trapped in follicles that do not respond to the LH surge and thus would degenerate.

RECEPTORS FOR OTHER HORMONES

Receptors for androgens[48], progestins[49], GnRH[50], and prolactin[51,52] have also been localized in rat granulosa cells. The precise roles of each of these hormones during follicular growth and the mechanisms regulating receptor number during granulosa cell differentiation in most cases await clarification. Androgens, for example, given *in vivo* to hypophysectomized oestradiol-treated rats (i.e. in the absence of gonadotrophins) cause rampant follicular atresia[53]. In contrast, when gonadotrophins are present (i.e. in the intact oestradiol-treated rat), androgens block FSH stimulated increases in LH receptor but do not exert major atretogenic effects[54,55]. Androgens added *in vitro* to granulosa cell cultures actually enhance FSH stimulation of progesterone accumulation[56,57] and do not cause granulosa cell death. Therefore, *in vivo*, LH-induced increases in androgen production may not only serve to provide a substrate for the aromatase enzyme system but also may act as a hormone to facilitate progesterone synthesis.

Progesterone is known to act on the hypothalamo-hypophyseal axis to inhibit gonadotrophin secretion. However, direct negative effects of progesterone on follicular tissue have also been proposed[58-60]. The results of studies using immature rats and progesterone implants strongly suggest that the primary effect of progesterone *in vivo* is to suppress LH secretion and inhibit the LH surge[28]. Nevertheless, very high concentrations of progesterone, such as those stimulated by the LH surge, may exert local inhibitory effects. Although progesterone does not act to decrease ovarian receptors for oestradiol[61] as it does in the uterus, progesterone does appear to inhibit aromatase activity[62].

GnRH and its agonists have been shown to inhibit FSH effects in rat granulosa cells, including induction of LH receptor, antrum formation and steroidogenesis[63]. Although the physiological GnRH remains to be identified it is possible that it plays a role in follicular atresia in the rat. The effects of GnRH are not as apparent in other species.

The role of prolactin in follicular development also remains ambiguous. While there is evidence that prolactin can exert negative effects on the function of granulosa cells in culture[52,64,65], there is other evidence from *in vivo* studies which suggests that prolactin also enhances ovarian activity in rats[66]. In women, hyperprolactinaemia is often associated with amenorrhoea. Fertility in most cases can be restored by reducing serum prolactin with ergot alkaloids[67].

In summary, the follicle is regulated by many different hormones, including steroids, proteins, glycoproteins and possibly small peptides. Our knowledge of the last group is scant but no doubt in the future other regulatory substances will be clearly identified and purified.

References

1. Pederson, T. and Peters, H. (1971). *Fertil. Steril.*, **22**, 42
2. Richards, J. S. (1980). *Physiol. Rev.*, **60**, 51
3. Oakberg, E. F. and Tyrell, P. D. (1975). *Biol. Reprod.*, **12**, 477
4. Pederson, T. (1970). *Acta Endocrinol. (Kbh)*, **64**, 304
5. Chiras, D. D. and Greenwald, G. S. (1977). *Anat. Rec.*, **188**, 331
6. Faddy, M. J., Jones, E. C. and Edwards, R. G. (1976). *J. Exp. Zool.*, **197**, 173
7. Hirshfield, A. N. and Midgley, A. R., Jr. (1978). *Biol. Reprod.*, **19**, 597
8. Butcher, R. L., Collins, W. E. and Fugo, N. W. (1974). *Endocrinology*, **94**, 1704
9. Gay, V. L., Midgley, A. R., Jr. and Niswender, G. D. (1970). *Fed. Proc.*, **29**, 1880
10. Smith, M. E., Freeman, M. E. and Neill, J. D. (1975). *Endocrinology*, **96**, 219
11. Morishige, W. K., Pepe, G. J. and Rothchild, I. (1973). *Endocrinology*, **92**, 1527
12. Bogovich, K. and Richards, J. S. (1981). *Endocrinology*, **109**, 860
13. Schwartz, N. B. (1974). *Reprod. Biol.*, **10**, 236
14. Welschen, R. (1973). *Acta Endocrinol. (Kbh)*, **72**, 137
15. Richards, J. S. and Kersey, K. A. (1979). *Biol. Reprod.*, **21**, 1185
16. Bates, R. W. and Schooley, J. P. (1942). *Endocrinology*, **31**, 309
17. Lostroh, A. J. and Johnson, R. E. (1966). *Endocrinology*, **79**, 991
18. Midgley, A. R., Jr. (1973). *Adv. Exp. Med. Biol.*, **36**, 365
19. Richards, J. S., Ireland, J. J., Rao, M. C., Bernath, G. A., Midgley, A. R., Jr. and Reichert, L. E., Jr. (1976). *Endocrinology*, **99**, 1562
20. Richards, J. S., Jonassen, J. A., Rolfes, A. I., Kersey, K. A. and Reichert, L. E., Jr. (1979). *Endocrinology*, **104**, 765
21. Rao, M. C., Richards, J. S. and Midgley, A. R., Jr. (1978). *Cell*, **14**, 71
22. Richards, J. S. and Rolfes, A. I. (1980). *J. Biol. Chem.*, **255**, 5481
23. Ireland, J. J. and Richards, J. S. (1978). *Endocrinology*, **102**, 876
24. Jonassen, J. A. and Richards, J. S. (1980). *Endocrinology*, **106**, 1786
25. Hunzicker-Dunn, M. and Birnbaumer, L. (1976). *Endocrinology*, **99**, 198
26. Rao, M. C., Richards, J. S., Midgley, A. R., Jr. and Reichert, L. E., Jr. (1977). *Endocrinology*, **101**, 512
27. Richards, J. S. (1979). *Recent Prog. Horm. Res.*, **35**, 343
28. Richards, J. S., Jonassen, J. A. and Kersey, K. A. (1980). *Endocrinology*, **107**, 641
29. Carson, R. S., Kahn, L. E. and Richards, J. S. (1981). *Endocrinology*, **109**, 1433
30. Karsch, F. J. (1980). *The Physiologist*, **23**, 29
31. Zeleznick, A. J., Midgley, A. R., Jr. and Reichert, L. E., Jr. (1974). *Endocrinology*, **95**, 818
32. Uilenbroek, J. Th. J. and Richards, J. S. (1979). *Biol. Reprod.*, **20**, 1159
33. Channing, C. P. and Kammerman, S. (1974). *Biol. Reprod.*, **10**, 179
34. Fortune, J. E. and Armstrong, D. T. (1977). *Endocrinology*, **100**, 1341
35. Pencharz, R. I. (1940). *Science*, **91**, 554
36. Williams, P. C. (1945). *J. Endocrinol.*, **4**, 127
37. Bradbury, J. T. (1961). *Endocrinology*, **68**, 115
38. Stumpf, W. E. (1969). *Endocrinology*, **85**, 31
39. Goldenberg, R. L., Vaitukaitis, J. L. and Ross, G. T. (1972). *Endocrinology*, **90**, 1492
40. Richards, J. S. (1975). *Endocrinology*, **97**, 1174
41. Richards, J. S. (1978). In Jones, R. E. (ed.) *Vertebrate Ovary*, p. 331. (New York: Plenum)
42. Gospodarowicz, D. S., Ill, C. R. and Birdwell, C. R. (1977). *Endocrinology*, **100**, 1108
43. Richards, J. S. and Midgley, A. R., Jr. (1976). *Biol. Reprod.*, **14**, 82
44. Marsh, J. M., Mills, T. M. and LeMaire, W. J. (1973). *Biochim. Biophys. Acta*, **304**, 197
45. Robison, G. A., Butcher, R. W. and Sutherland, E. W. (1968). *Ann. Rev. Biochem.*, **37**, 149
46. Knecht, M., Amsterdam, A. and Catt, K. (1981). *J. Biol. Chem.*, **256**, 10628
47. Jonassen, J. A., Bose, K. and Richards, J. S. (1984). *Endocrinology*, (In press)
48. Schreiber, J. R. and Ross, G. T. (1976). *Endocrinology*, **99**, 590
49. Schreiber, J. R. and Erickson, G. F. (1979). *Steroids*, **34**, 459
50. Pieper, D., Richards, J. S. and Marshall, J. (1981). *Endocrinology*, **108**, 1148
51. Richards, J. S. and Williams, J. J. (1976). *Endocrinology*, **99**, 1571
52. Hseuh, A. J. W., Wang, C. and Erickson, G. F. (1980). *Endocrinology*, **106**, 1679
53. Louvet, J.-P., Harman, S. M., Schreiber, J. R. and Ross, G. T. (1975). *Endocrinology*, **97**, 366
54. Farookhi, R. (1980). *Endocrinology*, **106**, 1216
55. Farookhi, R. (1981). In Schwartz, N. B. and Hunzicker-Dunn, M. (eds.) *Dynamics of Ovarian Function*, p. 13. (New York: Raven Press)

56. Lucky, A. W., Schreiber, J. R., Hillier, S. G., Schulman, J. D. and Ross, G. T. (1977). *Endocrinology*, **100**, 128
57. Nimrod, A. and Lindner, H. R. (1976). *Mol. Cell Endocrinol.*, **5**, 315
58. Kalra, S. P. and Kalra, P. S. (1974). *Endocrinology*, **95**, 1711
59. Greenwald, G. S. (1977). *J. Endocrinol.*, **73**, 151
60. Hess, D. L. and Resko, J. A. (1973). *Endocrinology*, **92**, 446
61. Saiddudin, S. and Zassenhaus, H. P. (1978). *Endocrinology*, **102**, 1069
62. Schreiber, J. R., Nakamura, K. and Erickson, G. F. (1981). In Schwartz, N. B. and Hunzicker-Dunn, M. (eds.) *Dynamics of Ovarian Function*, p. 67. (New York: Raven Press)
63. Wang, C., Hseuh, A. J. W. and Erickson, G. F. (1979). *J. Biol. Chem.*, **254**, 11330
64. Dorrington, J. H. and Gore-Langton, R. E. (1982). *Endocrinology*, **110**, 1701
65. McNatty, K. P. (1979). *Fertil. Steril.*, **32**, 433
66. Advis, J. P., Richards, J. S. and Ojeda, S. R. (1981). *Endocrinology*, **108**, 1333
67. Bohnet, H. C. and McNeilly, A. S. (1979). *Horm. Metab. Res.*, **11**, 533

3
Recruitment, selection and maturation of the dominant ovarian follicle in the menstrual cycle

G. D. Hodgen

In recent reviews[1–3] we have described ongoing follicular, ovulatory and luteal events of the adult ovary during the primate menstrual cycle. Much less attention has been given to factors regulating the initiation of cyclic ovarian function; that is, the establishment of normal ovulation beyond the perimenarchial and postpartum intervals. Because some similarities exist in the initiation of cyclic ovarian function during puberty and after pregnancy-induced anovulation in both women and monkeys, we have studied both the initiation and restoration of cyclic ovarian activity during the menarche and postpartum, respectively[4].

The establishment of folliculogenesis culminating in ovulation and normal corpus luteum function, with the potential of initiation and supporting pregnancy, is an end-point achieved only after the gradual integration of the hypothalamic–pituitary–ovarian axis. This scenario includes neuronal signals emanating from beyond the medial–basal hypothalamus for the provision of intermittent GnRH release[5], appropriate FSH and LH secretion from the anterior pituitary—including the modulation of FSH:LH ratios[6,7] and the biopotency of certain molecular entities of these glycoprotein hormones[8,9], as well as the institution of both negative and positive feedback (steroidal or non-steroidal) from the ovaries upon processes governing the synthesis and secretion of pituitary gonadotrophins[10–13].

DEFINITION OF TERMS

A brief review of specific terms used here may help communicate our meaning (Figure 1). *Recruitment* is a process whereby a follicle(s) begins to mature in a milieu of sufficient pituitary gonadotrophic stimulation to permit progress toward ovulation; a cohort may be of N size. *Selection* is the process by which typically a single follicle is chosen; ultimately, it alone may avoid atresia and is competent to achieve timely ovulation. Among women and these monkeys, asymmetrical ovarian function is inherent to maturation of the dominant follicle. *Dominance* is the means by which the selected (dominant) follicle, or its successor

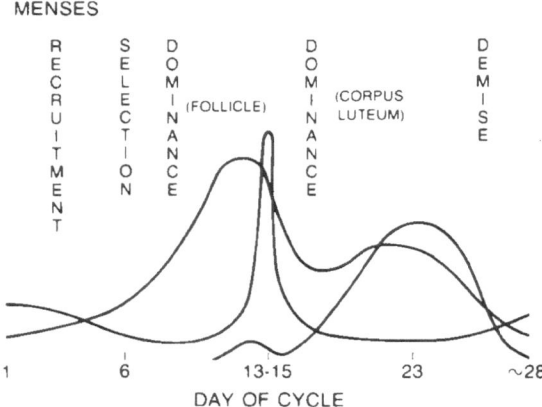

Figure 1 The terms used to describe the sequence of principal ovarian events during follicular maturation and corpus luteum function are temporally defined in the menstrual cycle. The curves depict idealized (typical) patterns of oestradiol, pituitary gonadotrophins and progesterone in peripheral circulation

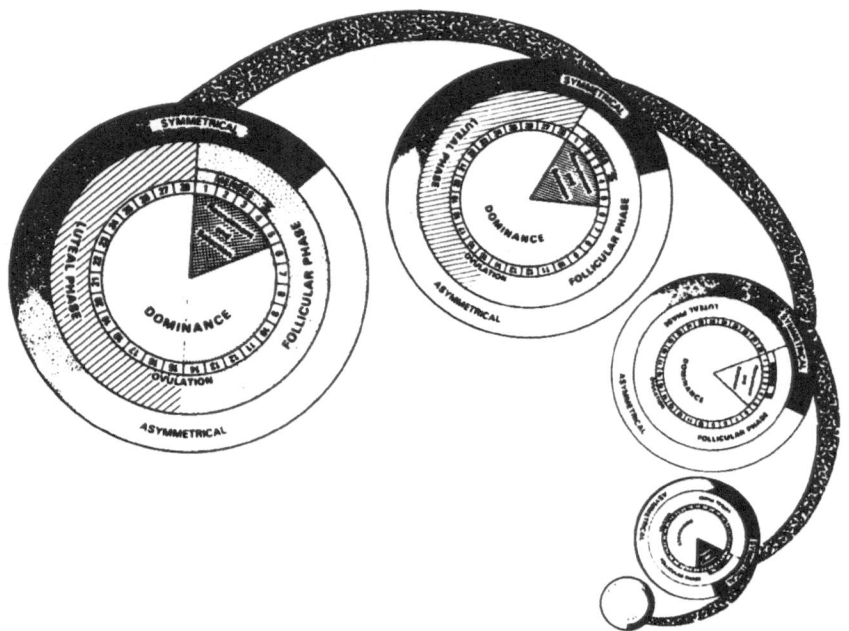

Figure 2 Composite conceptualization of the primate ovarian/menstrual cycle summarizing work presented throughout this review (Reproduced with permission from reference 2.)

the corpus luteum, maintains its eminence bilaterally over all other follicles, dictating the course of events in the hypothalamus, pituitary, and the ovaries both temporally and spatially for the duration of that same menstrual cycle. *Demise* of the corpus luteum ends the reigning influence of this antecedent dominant structure. Thus, in the absence of maternal recognition of pregnancy (fertile menstrual cycle), the ovarian and menstrual cycles are renewed concurrently after respective follicular and luteal phases over sequential fortnightly courses (Figure 2).

THE FOLLICULAR POOL

Any ovarian follicle destined to ovulate is derived from a cohort of growing follicles drawn, in turn, from a pool of non-proliferating primordial follicles formed during fetal development (Figure 3). We know that pituitary gonadotrophins support this progression of follicular maturation[2] and that about 99.9% of all ovarian follicles are lost spontaneously to atresia; only an exceptional few achieve ovulation (Figure 4). It is not clear how the ovulatory quota is determined. Depending on the species, typically only a few or even just one of these follicles of a given cohort escape atresia at various stages of development and finally reach maturity, culminating in ovulation of a fertilizable oocyte. This successive reduction of potentially ovulatory follicles during each ovarian cycle

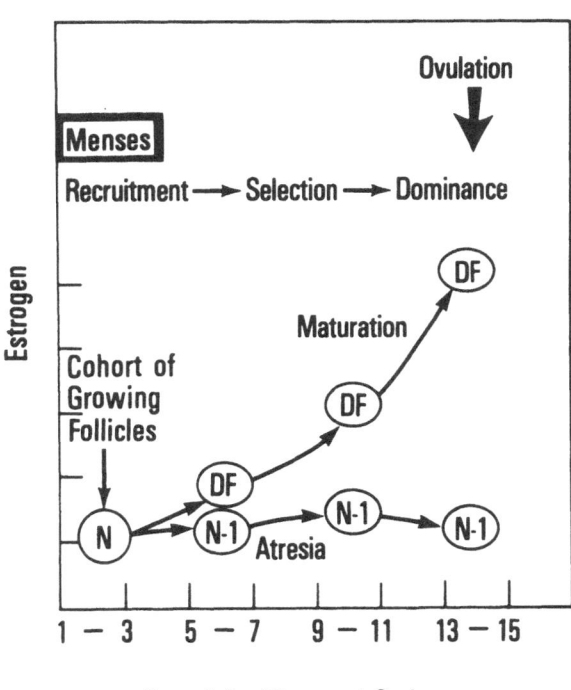

Figure 3 Time course for recruitment and selection of the dominant follicle with onset of atresia among other follicles of the cohort

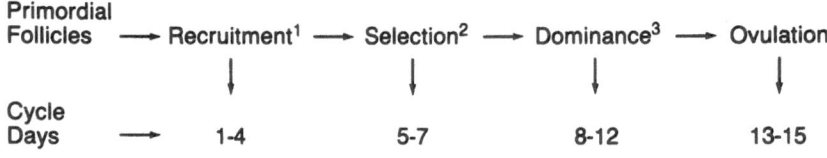

Definitions:

1 = Cohort May be: N = 1 or N = >1

2 = A Single Follicle is Destined to Ovulate;
No Surrogate Follicles

3 = Dominance May be:

Active = Dominant Follicle Suppresses
Maturation of Other Follicles

Passive = Dominant Follicle Thrives Uniquely,
Despite the Suppressive Milieu

Figure 4 The cohort of follicles from which the ovulatory follicle is derived begins to grow about day 1 of the menstrual cycle. The number of follicles in a cohort is unknown, but is typically reduced to the ovulatory quota (unity) during the mid-follicular phase

to a number characteristic of the species implies some process of selection. This is especially evident in the higher primates, including women, where typically the process of folliculogenesis, leading to the elaboration of a single mature gamete in each menstrual cycle, is regulated with a high degree of precision.

Among the salient issues in understanding the regulation of follicle growth is to learn what determines whether a follicle will remain at rest, develop and ovulate, or become atretic. Folliculogenesis is the result of three constituent processes of the follicle: rest (latency) and then growth culminating in ovulation or, more often, atresia. Consequently, to study the regulation of folliculogenesis is to uncover the mechanism(s) that determines in which developmental stage a follicle will be found.

We began by asking a series of principal questions:

(1) What is the *time course* of new follicle growth?
(2) When is the dominant follicle *selected*?
(3) How is *dominance* maintained, so that a single follicle is ovulated?
(4) If the dominant follicle fails, when is it replaced by *new follicle growth*?
(5) How many follicles are *recruited* into growth?
(6) How do pituitary *gonadotrophins* participate in the regulation of follicle growth?
(7) What determines the *location* of new follicle growth, between and within the ovaries?

DURATION OF THE MATURATIONAL SEQUENCE

Having imposed a sudden interruption of the ovarian cycle by ablating the 'cyclic structure' (either dominant follicle or corpus luteum), we found that after ablation of the largest visible follicle, the expected midcycle surges of oestradiol, LH, and FSH were abolished, with the next preovulatory surges occurring 12–14 days after cautery[14]. These surges were indistinguishable from those typifying a normal menstrual cycle. Only a single follicle ovulated and luteinized in each monkey; the ovulatory quota was not affected. The secretory activity and lifespan of the new corpus luteum were typical of normal cycles. Moreover, circulating levels of gonadotrophins were maintained after follicle cautery until the next preovulatory surges.

These results indicated that cautery of the largest follicle destroyed the follicle destined to ovulate since the expected surges of oestradiol and gonadotrophin secretion did not occur at midcycle but were delayed by about 2 weeks. Since this delay approximated the length of a typical follicular phase, it appeared that no other follicle(s) was competent to substitute for the cauterized follicle to accommodate a timely ovulation. Instead, the delay suggested that the follicle destined to ovulate had been selected already by the day of cautery, that is, by the mid-follicular phase, and that the next follicle to ovulate was the product of a new cohort of one or more follicles that developed after cautery.

That the interval between luteectomy and the next LH surge was of the same duration as that after follicle cautery indicates that interruption at either phase of the cycle is followed by a similar response. Thus, the ovarian steroidal milieu at the time of ablation did not seem to affect the response. Otherwise, the response to ablation in the luteal phase, after midcycle surges had occurred, would presumably have been different from the response to cautery in the follicular phase, before the midcycle surges had occurred. Moreover, midcycle surges of oestradiol and gonadotrophins are not required to initiate preovulatory follicular maturation[1,14]. Recently, these findings were confirmed after ablation of the dominant follicle or corpus luteum in women[15].

Therefore, based on these findings, we reasoned that: (1) new follicle growth during the monkey's ovarian cycle is arrested in the presence of the dominant follicle or corpus luteum; (2) gonadotrophins are necessary, but not sufficient to support follicular maturation leading to ovulatory status; and (3) the dominant follicle and corpus luteum seemed to inhibit follicle growth at the level of the ovaries, since after ablation of these cyclic structures, follicle growth resumed anew, seemingly more as a result of a local disinhibition than from a compensatory increase in gonadotrophic stimulation. Clearly, the dominant follicle and the corpus luteum comprise the 'dominant structures' of the ovarian cycle, having remarkable authority over both intraovarian (bilateral) and systemic events regulating folliculogenesis.

THE INTEROVARIAN PROGESTERONE GRADIENT

Our experience indicates that the side of ovulation in monkeys is neither completely random nor repetitively alternating. That is, the next ovulation occurs contralateral to the corpus luteum about 70% of the time in normal, unperturbed menstrual cycles. Accordingly, the interovarian progesterone gradient dissipates gradually during the spontaneous demise of the corpus luteum in the late luteal phase of the non-fertile menstrual cycle. Although follicles in the ovary contralateral to the antecedent ovulation have an apparent relative advantage for recruitment in the subsequent cycle, perhaps by virtue of lower intraovarian progesterone, this facility is not absolute[16–18]. Indeed, some (fewer) follicles in the ipsilateral ovary may avoid antagonism by progesterone concurrent with the passing corpus luteum, therein manifesting full responsivity to the factors which promote timely selection and ovulation of the next dominant follicle.

On the basis of the foregoing series of investigations, we have concluded that intraovarian progesterone probably is a principal determinant of new follicle growth, regulating selection of the dominant follicle both spatially and temporally in the primate menstrual cycle.

RENEWAL OF THE OVARIAN CYCLE

The increase in circulating FSH typically associated with the spontaneous demise of the corpus luteum during the antecedent luteal phase and approximately the interval of menses in the subsequent follicular phases of women[6] and monkeys[19] has been regarded as potentially significant for follicular recruitment in the subsequent primate ovarian cycle. We doubt the surety of this interpretation: if timely recruitment, selection and maturation of the dominant follicle are dependent on hormonal events of an antecedent cycle, such as the midcycle gonadotrophin surges or the intercycle FSH elevation (Figure 5), how could the *first ovulation* be achieved—either in the postmenarchial interval or after the gestational hiatus of cyclic ovarian function in the postpartum months?

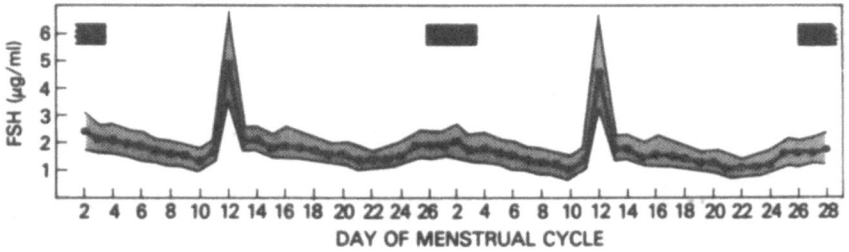

Figure 5   The intercycle FSH elevation is the peripheral serum FSH rise beginning during the late luteal phase and extending through the interval of menses into the next follicular phase (Reproduced with permission from reference 2.)

We investigated the significance of the intercycle serum FSH elevation in the primate ovarian cycle by serial cautery of the largest visible follicle (the putative dominant follicle) during the preovulatory interval (about cycle day 10) in two consecutive cycles[20]. In the third cycle, folliculogenesis was not disturbed and the spontaneous ovulation, 13–15 days after the second follicle cautery, was accompanied by normal follicular and luteal phase patterns of serum LH, FSH, oestradiol, and progesterone, including the usual rise in the late luteal phase (intercycle) FSH levels.

These findings indicated that the late luteal phase elevation in serum FSH is not obligatory for timely recruitment and selection of the subsequent dominant follicle. Further, despite ablation of the dominant follicle in two consecutive ovarian cycles, no surrogate follicles were immediately competent to replace the dominant follicle, and timely new follicle growth continued in a third follicular phase without a significant increase in mean circulating FSH, although post-ablative FSH patterns were more variable than normal. Thus, timely recruitment, selection and ovulation of the dominant follicle can continue without an antecedent FSH increase like that which normally develops in the late luteal phase. These results in monkeys do not imply that serum FSH levels have little significance in folliculogenesis. On the contrary, FSH in synergism with oestrogen and LH is known to be directly responsible for follicular maturation[21]. Indeed, in both women[22] and monkeys[7, 23], subnormal FSH and oestradiol levels during the early follicular phase have been associated with dysfunctions of the corpus luteum in the subsequent luteal phase[3].

THE ASYMMETRY OF OVARIAN FUNCTION

Despite perfusion of both ovaries with the same peripheral blood and, therefore, similar exposure to pituitary gonadotrophins, typically only one of the two primate ovaries sponsors recruitment and selection of the single dominant follicle destined for ovulation later in the same cycle, usually about 14 days after the onset of menses. Random comparisons of sex steroid hormone levels in venous effluent from the two ovaries and in peripheral venous blood during ovulatory cycles have shown that both ovaries produce steroids throughout the cycle, but once a dominant follicle was overtly identifiable, levels of oestrogens, androgens and progestogens were dramatically elevated in the venous effluent from the ovary containing that follicle[24]. Indeed, rising steroid hormone levels in women and monkeys occur coincident with the rapid preovulatory growth of the dominant follicle in the late follicular phase[3].

Accordingly, we asked the questions: when in the follicular phase of the primate ovarian cycle does ovarian function become asymmetrical, as determined from steroid hormones secreted into the ovarian venous effluent; and do these early hormonal indices of asymmetry reliably foretell the locus of the coming dominant follicle? By sequentially sampling ovarian venous effluents after the spontaneous onset of menses[25], we found that oestradiol levels in ovarian vein blood became asymmetrical 5–7 days before the midcycle gonadotrophin surge, or in a related protocol by 5 days after luteectomy[25]. Not surprisingly, the degree of asymmetry increased with progression toward ovulation (Figure 6). In each case, the ovary secreting the higher oestradiol concentration early on was later found to contain the functional corpus luteum. Disparate secretions of androstenedione and progesterone were not evident until 2–3 days before the midcycle FSH/LH surge. Whether this early initiation of asymmetrical secretion of ovarian oestradiol constitutes expression of dominance of one ovary, from which the dominant follicle ultimately arises, or whether the selected follicle itself is responsible for this early asymmetry of ovarian performance is unknown. Asymmetrical ovarian oestrogen secretion may be among the earliest indicators that the dominant follicle, or at least the ovary destined to bear it, typically is selected at midfollicular phase[24]. In fact, we uniformly found clear-cut disparity of oestradiol secretion by cycle days 5–7 unless the cycle in progress was destined to be anovulatory.

These findings establish that although several large antral follicles, contemporaneous with the authentic dominant follicle, arise and persist bilaterally into the late follicular phase in both women and monkeys, apparently these follicles

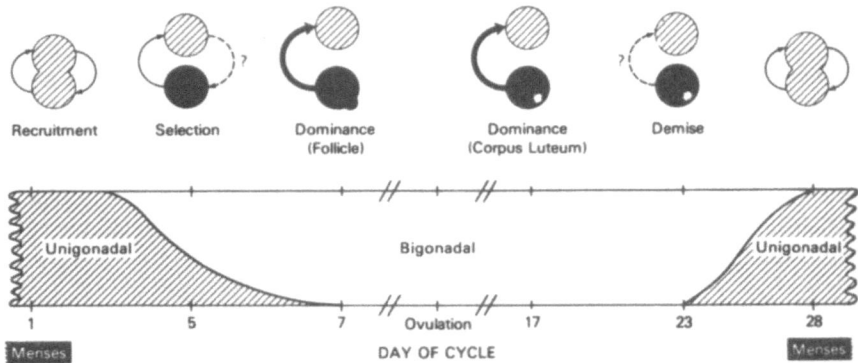

Figure 6 Transient nature of asymmetrical ovarian function in the primate menstrual/ovarian cycle. The terms unigonadal and bigonadal may be used interchangeably with symmetrical and asymmetrical, respectively (Reproduced with permission from reference 2.)

contribute little to oestradiol, androstenedione, or progesterone levels in ovarian vein blood[24]. It has generally been thought that a follicle containing high concentrations of oestrogens in its follicular fluid may also secrete large amounts of oestradiol into ovarian venous blood. However, some studies have suggested that not all such follicles are functionally active. Indeed, others[26] have shown that high levels of androgens in human follicular fluid correlated with morphological signs of follicular atresia. Moreover, since the overt dominant follicle has no surrogates soon competent to replace it[15,24], these several large antral follicles may have been predestined to atresia.

PULSATILE SECRETION OF BIOASSAYABLE LH

Dynamic changes in pulsatile gonadotrophin secretion accompanied the initiation of the preovulatory FSH and LH surges in the late follicular phase[27]. Prodigious elevations of bioassayable LH develop within 24 h (Figure 7). Further, the data suggested that the ascending limb of the bioassayable LH surge began to rise 4–6 h prior to a discernible onset of the surge mode of LH and FSH secretion measured by radioimmunoassay[8]. As the disparity between the bioassayable versus immunoassayable LH grew, the B:I ratio rose to as much as 10:1. The greater amplitude of bioassayable LH pulses was particularly evident in the establishment of the preovulatory surge. Similarly, bioassayable LH returned to tonic levels severals hours later than immunoassayable LH[9].

These findings establish that the pulsatile secretion of bioassayable LH undergoes a transition from the tonic mode to the surge mode in a manner that is temporally, quantitatively and qualitatively distinct from immunoassayable LH[8], as assessed in these assay systems. The enhanced biological activity of LH during the surge mode of secretion may have significance, previously under-appreciated, in synchronizing final maturation of the preovulatory follicle and the ovum. We expect that the degree of disparity between bioassayable LH and immuno-assayable LH will depend very much on the binding characteristics of the antisera used in various radioimmunoassays.

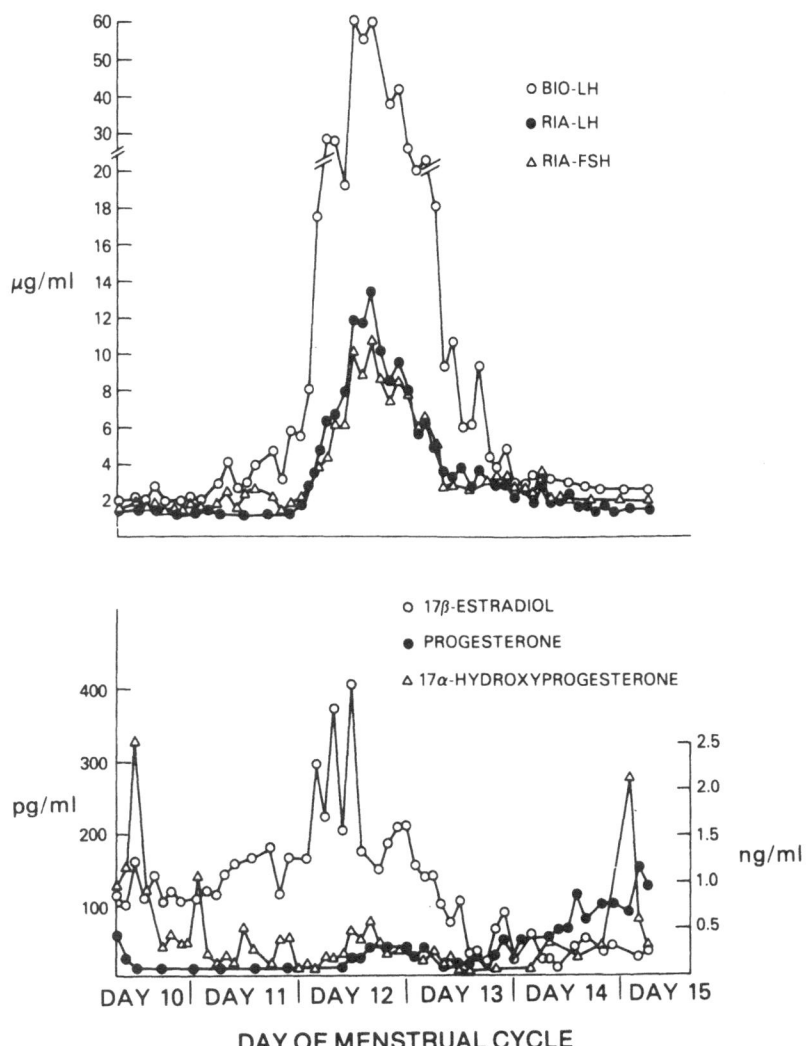

Figure 7 Periovulatory patterns of principal ovarian steroids and pituitary gonadotrophins in a rhesus monkey. Note disparity of BIO-LH and RIA-LH curves (LER 1909–2 standard) during the preovulatory surge (blood collected at 2-hour intervals)

COLLECTING THE OVUM BY FOLLICULAR ASPIRATION

The antrum of the preovulatory follicle contains the ovum, as well as follicular fluid and granulosa cells[28]. This special milieu is unique to the mature dominant follicle, being rich in chemical constituents as yet incompletely characterized. In this environment, the oocyte extrudes excess nuclear material in final preparation for fertilization. These events occur in the last hours of the follicular phase, almost during the ovulatory process.

DISRUPTION OF LUTEAL FUNCTION

As mentioned previously, there are potentially damaging sequelae to the surgical removal of the ovum from the preovulatory follicle[29]. When the egg is collected from the antrum, unavoidably, follicular fluid and granulosa cells are removed as well. Thus, essential biochemical interactions occurring within the gamete and surrounding ovarian support cells may be interrupted.

When multiple follicular maturation has been induced through administration of exogenous hormones, a strategy being applied widely now for *in vitro* fertilization[30–32], the collective secretions of more than one corpus luteum may ameliorate the threat of luteal-phase hormonal deficiency. Even so, it must be realized that whatever aberrancies of folliculogenesis accompany exogenous hormonal therapy, given to increase the number of ova available, will be added to the consequences of follicular aspiration on the ovum, corpus luteum and endometrial normalcy[28].

Acknowledgments

I appreciate the outstanding efforts of the entire technical research staff of the Pregnancy Research Branch, as well as the creative and tireless endeavours of the following postdoctoral fellows: Doctors Goodman, Stouffer, Williams, diZerega, Kreitmann, Marut, and Schenken. Also, I am grateful for the skills of Ms Linda Baldwin in preparing this manuscript.

References

1. diZerega, G. S. and Hodgen, G. D. (1980). Changing functional status of the monkey corpus luteum. *Biol. Reprod.*, **23**, 253
2. diZerega, G. S. and Hodgen, G. D. (1981). Folliculogenesis in the primate ovarian cycle. *Endocr. Rev.*, **2**, 27–49
3. diZerega, G. S. and Hodgen, G. D. (1981). Luteal phase dysfunction infertility: a sequel to aberrant folliculogenesis. *Fertil. Steril.*, **35**, 489–99
4. Williams, R. F. and Hodgen, G. D. (1982). Initiation of the primate ovarian cycle with emphasis on perimenarchial and postpartum events. In Greep (ed.) *Reproductive Physiology*. Vol. IV, pp. 1–55. (Baltimore: University Park Press)
5. Knobil, E. (1980). The neuroendocrine control of the menstrual cycle. *Rec. Prog. Horm. Res.*, **36**, 53
6. Ross, G. T., Cargille, C. M., Lipsett, M. B., *et al.* (1970). Pituitary and gonadal induced ovulatory cycles. *Rec. Prog. Horm. Res.*, **26**, 1
7. Wilks, J. W., Hodgen, G. D. and Ross, G. T. (1976). Luteal phase defects in the rhesus monkey: the significance of serum FSH:LH ratios. *J. Clin. Endocrinol. Metab.*, **43**, 1261–8
8. Marut, E. L., Williams, R. F., Cowan, B. D., Lynch, A., Lerner, S. P. and Hodgen, G. D. (1981). Pulsatile pituitary gonadotropin secretion during maturation of the dominant follicle in monkeys: estrogen positive feedback enhances the biological activity of LH. *Endocrinology*, **109**, 2270–2
9. Williams, R. F., Turner, C. K. and Hodgen, G. D. (1982). The late pubertal cascade in perimenarchial monkeys: onset of asymmetrical ovarian estradiol secretion and bioassayable LH release. *J. Clin. Endocrinol. Metab.*, **55**, 660–5
10. Dierschke, D. J., Weiss, G. and Knobil, E. (1974). Sexual maturation in the female rhesus monkey and the development of estrogen-induced gonadotropic hormone release. *Endocrinology*, **94**, 198
11. Goodman, A. L. and Hodgen, G. D. (1978). Post partum patterns of circulating FSH, LH, prolactin, estradiol and progesterone in nonsuckling cynomolgus monkeys. *Steroids*, **31**, 731
12. Rebar, R. W. and Yen, S. S. C. (1979). Endocrine rhythms in gonadotropin and ovarian steroids with reference to reproductive processes. In Kreiger, D. T. (ed.) *Endocrine Rhythms*. p. 259. (New York: Raven Press)
13. Williams, R. F., Johnson, D. K. and Hodgen, G. D. (1979). Resumption of estrogen-induced gonadotropin surges in postpartum monkeys. *J. Clin. Endocrinol. Metab.*, **49**, 422

14. Goodman, A. L., Nixon, W. E., Johnson, D. L. and Hodgen, G. D. (1977). Regulation of folliculogenesis in the rhesus monkey: selection of the dominant follicle. *Endocrinology*, **100**, 155–63
15. Nilsson, L., Wikland, M. and Hamberger, L. (1982). Recruitment of and ovulatory follicle in the human following follicle-ectomy and luteectomy. *Fertil. Steril.*, **37**, 30–4
16. Goodman, A. L. and Hodgen, G. D. (1977). Systemic versus intraovarian progesterone replacement after luteectomy in rhesus monkeys: differential patterns of gonadotropins and follicle growth. *J. Clin. Endocrinol. Metab.*, **45**, 837–43
17. Goodman, A. L. and Hodgen, G. D. (1979). Between-ovary interaction in the regulation of follicle growth, corpus luteum function and gonadotropin secretion in the primate ovarian cycle II. Effects of luteectomy and hemiovariectomy during the luteal phase in cynomolgus monkeys. *Endocrinology*, **104**, 1310–18
18. diZerega, G. S. and Hodgen, G. D. (1982). The interovarian progesterone gradient: a spatial and temporal regulator of folliculogenesis in the primate ovarian cycle. *J. Clin. Endocrinol. Metab.*, **54**, 495–9
19. Hodgen, G. D., Wilks, J. W., Vaitukaitis, J. L., Chen, H. C., Papkoff, H. and Ross, G. T. (1976). A new radioimmunoassay for follicle stimulating hormone in macaques: ovulatory menstrual cycles. *Endocrinology*, **99**, 137–46
20. diZerega, G. S., Nixon, W. E. and Hodgen, G. D. (1980). Intercycle serum FSH elevations: significance in recruitment and selection of the dominant follicle and assessment of corpus luteum normalcy. *J. Clin. Endocrinol. Metab.*, **50**, 1046–8
21. Richards, J. S. (1979). Hormonal control of follicular growth and maturation in mammals. In Jones, R. E. (ed.) *The Vertebrate Ovary*. p. 331. (New York: Plenum Press)
22. Jones, G. S. (1976). The luteal phase defect. *Fertil. Steril.*, **27**, 351
23. Stouffer, R. L. and Hodgen, G. D. (1980). Induction of luteal phase defects in rhesus monkeys by follicular fluid administration at the onset of the menstrual cycle. *J. Clin. Endocrinol. Metab.*, **51**, 669–71
24. diZerega, G. S., Marut, E. L., Turner, C. K. and Hodgen, G. D. (1980). Asymmetrical ovarian function during recruitment and selection of the dominant follicle in the menstrual cycle of the rhesus monkey. *J. Clin. Endocrinol. Metab.*, **51**, 698–701
25. diZerega, G. S. and Hodgen, G. D. (1981). Initiation of asymmetrical ovarian estradiol secretion in the primate ovarian cycle after luteectomy. *Endocrinology*, **108**, 1233–6
26. McNatty, K. P., Smith, D. M., Makris, A., Osathanondh, R. and Ryan, K. J. (1979). The microenvironment of the human antral follicle: interrelationships among the steroid levels in antral fluid, the population of granulosa cells, and the status of the oocyte *in vivo* and *in vitro*. *J. Clin. Endocrinol. Metab.*, **49**, 851, 611–12
27. Schenken, R. S., Cowan, B. D., Sopelak, V. M., Williams, R. F. and Hodgen, G. D. (1982). Periovulatory patterns of principal ovarian steroids and pituitary gonadotropins in monkeys with and without a trapped ovum. *Fertil. Steril.*, **40**
28. Hodgen, G. D. (1981). *In vitro* fertilization and alternatives. *J. Am. Med. Assoc.*, **246**, 590–7
29. Kreitmann, O. and Hodgen, G. D. (1981). Induced corpus luteum dysfunction after aspiration of the preovulatory follicle in monkeys. *Fertil. Steril.*, **35**, 671–5
30. Edwards, R. G., Steptoe, P. C. and Purdy, J. M. (1980). Establishing full-term human pregnancies using cleaving embryos grown *in vitro*. *Br. J. Obstet. Gynaecol.*, **87**, 737–56
31. Wood, C., Trounson, A., Leeton, J., *et al.* (1981). A clinical assessment of nine pregnancies obtained by *in vitro* fertilization and embryo transfer. *Fertil. Steril.*, **35**, 502–9
32. Jones, H. W., Acosta, A. A. and Garcia, J. (1982). A technique for the aspiration of oocytes from human ovarian follicles. *Fertil. Steril.*, **37**, 26–9

4
Intraovarian regulation of maturation of granulosa cells

C. P. Channing, M. R. Loeken, K. G. Osteen and S. J. Atlas

DESCRIPTION OF GRANULOSA CELL MATURATION

Early during their maturation, the granulosa cells of small antral follicles contain numerous receptors for follicle stimulating hormone (FSH), but very few for luteinizing hormone (LH)[1]. Presumably by stimulating cAMP accumulation, FSH activates several processes in granulosa cells, the best studied being aromatization of androgens to oestrogens[2], induction of LH receptors [3–5] and increased ability to synthesize and secrete progesterone[5,6]. Aromatase enzyme activity appears to decline as increased progesterone secretory activity is acquired, whether or not cells are exposed to gonadotrophins[7]. In addition to its peripheral effects, oestrogen (primarily oestradiol) modulates FSH effects on granulosa cells as discussed below. Some of these changes which occur in the porcine granulosa cells during follicular maturation are shown in Figure 1.

During follicular maturation, granulosa cells exhibit a 50–100-fold increase in number of LH receptors[10,12]. FSH has been demonstrated *in vitro* to induce LH receptors in granulosa cells from several mammalian species[3–5]. The mechanism by which this induction occurs is not known; however, experiments with porcine granulosa cells from our laboratory have shown that 48 h are required to observe increased hCG binding and that inhibition of protein synthesis with puromycin attenuates FSH induction of LH receptors[13–15]. These results would be consistent with FSH stimulating expression of the gene(s) coding for the LH receptor. It is critical that granulosa cells acquire LH receptors in order to respond to LH and allow for ovulation and proper luteinization.

ROLE OF GONADOTROPHINS AND STEROIDS IN INDUCTION OF GRANULOSA CELL MATURATION

The ability of granulosa cells to respond to gonadotrophins with increased progesterone secretion is also induced by FSH[4–6]. Although low levels of progesterone are secreted *in vitro* in the absence of hormones, FSH stimulation is necessary for optimum progesterone secretion in response to either FSH or LH.

45

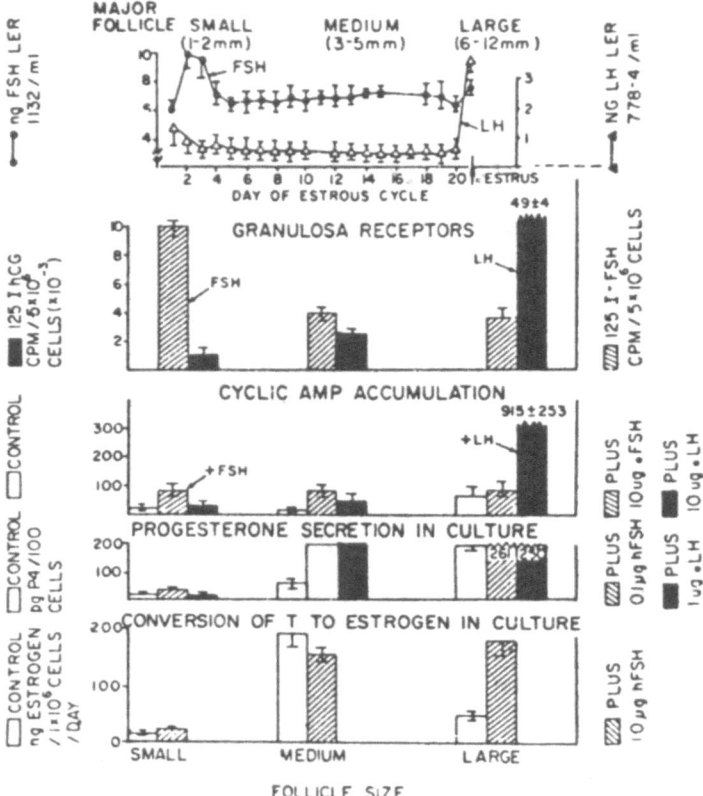

Figure 1 Changes occurring in porcine granulosa cells during follicular maturation. Data at the top represent serum FSH and LH levels occurring throughout the porcine oestrous cycle. Levels of FSH are adapted from the data of Rayford et al.[8] and levels of serum LH are adapted from the data of Niswender et al.[9]. Data on granulosa FSH binding are taken from Nakano et al.[43] and data on hCG binding are taken from Channing and Kammerman[10]. Data represent the mean $\pm$ SE of 6–15 observations. Data on the ability of FSH and LH to stimulate intracellular cyclic AMP accumulation represent the mean $\pm$ SE of 6–11 observations and are taken from Lindsey and Channing[11]. Observations on the effect of $1 \mu g \, ml^{-1}$ human FSH (LER 1801-3) and $1.0 \mu g \, ml^{-1}$ ovine LH on progesterone secretion are taken from the data of Thanki and Channing[6] using observations on granulosa cells cultured for 4 days (Taken from Channing et al.[44] with permission.)

Since at least 18 h of culture are required before detectable progesterone accumulates and inhibition of protein synthesis early in culture inhibits progesterone secretion, FSH may also stimulate expression of the genes governing progesterone synthesis and secretion[13-15].

These maturational changes in granulosa cells appear to take place under FSH stimulation to permit optimum responsiveness to the preovulatory LH surge; LH then induces ovulation and luteinization. In the co-ordinately matured granulosa cell, LH is a potent stimulator of cellular functions characteristic of luteal tissue such as progesterone secretion.

In addition to their peripheral effects, steroids produced during follicular maturation also have local effects within the ovary. Oestradiol has been demonstrated to be mitogenic to granulosa cells *in vivo*[16]. Oestrogen has also been found to modify gonadotrophin stimulated progesterone secretion. In many large mammals inhibition of progesterone secretion by granulosa or luteal cells occurs following exposure to oestradiol[6,17-20]. However, in the rat, and after several days of culture of highly differentiated porcine granulosa cells, oestradiol appears to potentiate progesterone secretion[21,22].

We have examined the effects of oestradiol with FSH on induction of the LH receptor, LH responsive cAMP accumulation and progesterone secretion by porcine granulosa cells during 4 days of culture. In a previous report we found that oestradiol does not inhibit, but appears to potentiate, FSH-stimulated induction of the LH receptor during 4 days of culture[13]. Similar data are shown in Figure 2. LH-responsive cAMP production was also not inhibited by oestradiol treatment (Figure 3). In contrast, progesterone secretion was inhibited by cells exposed to both oestradiol alone and oestradiol plus FSH (Figure 4). Thus, it appears that oestradiol inhibits progesterone secretion at some site distal to cAMP accumulation, perhaps at the level of protein kinase synthesis or activity, or progesterone synthetic or metabolic enzyme activity. The apparent potentiation of LH receptor induction by oestradiol may be important for optimum maturation of granulosa cells; inhibition of progesterone secretion may prevent premature luteinization of the follicle to maintain the proper synchrony of events during a fertile cycle.

It was also of interest to examine the effects of androgens on maturation of granulosa cells. In addition to serving as substrate for oestrogen biosynthesis, androgens have been implicated as either a cause or result of atresia since the androgen:oestrogen ratio has been found to be elevated in atretic follicles compared with healthy follicles[23]. Additionally, there is some evidence in the rat that androgens may inhibit the induction of functional LH receptors[24] which

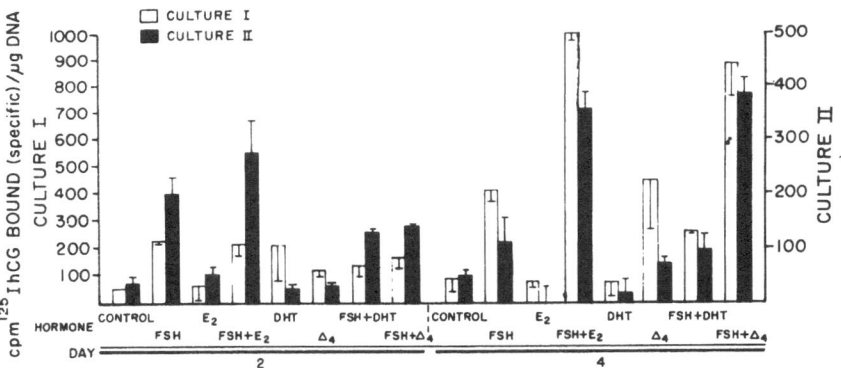

Figure 2 Influence of various hormone treatments upon specific [^{125}I]hCG binding of porcine granulosa cells after 2 and 4 days of culture. Data are from two separate series of granulosa cell cultures derived from different batches of porcine ovaries. Data are plotted separately and represent specific binding (total binding minus non-specific binding) $\pm$ SE derived from the SEM of total and non-specific binding values. The granulosa cells used for these cultures and those shown in Figures 3 and 4 were harvested from small (1–2 mm) porcine follicles

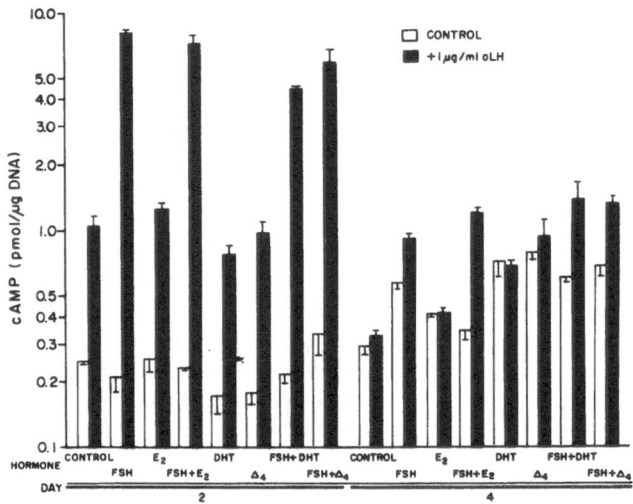

Figure 3 Influence of hormone treatments upon cyclic AMP production by porcine granulosa cells after 2 and 4 days of culture. The cultured granulosa cells were removed from the culture wells and challenged for 1 h with or without 1 μg ml^{-1} NIH ovine LH. Data are from one series of cultures obtained from one batch of porcine ovaries and represent the sum of cytoplasmic and secreted cAMP ± SE derived from the SEM of cytoplasmic and secreted values assayed in duplicate. Cyclic AMP was assayed in duplicate by radioimmunoassay (New England Nuclear)

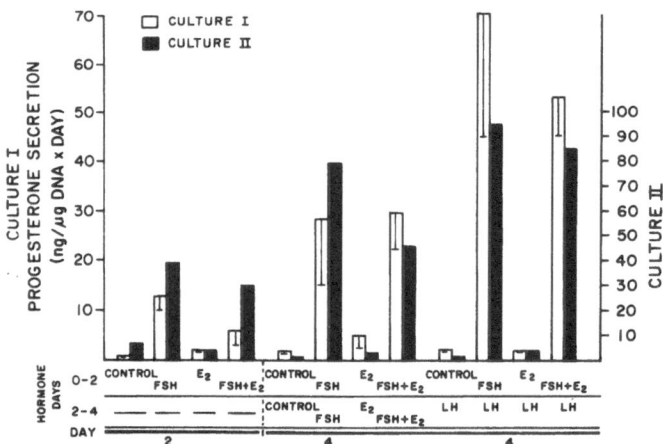

Figure 4 Influence of hormone treatments upon progesterone secretion during 2 and 4 days of culture. Media were aspirated from culture wells and saved for radioimmunoassay. Data are from two series of cultures in which two replicate culture wells per hormone treatment were assayed separately (Culture I) or one set of culture wells per hormone treatment was assayed (Culture II)

contrasts with the observation that androgens may synergize with FSH on progestin production[25]. Preliminary evidence from our laboratory suggests that during 4 days of culture of porcine granulosa cells, neither dihydrotestosterone (a non-aromatizable androgen), nor androstenedione (an aromatizable androgen) inhibit LH receptor induction or LH-responsive cAMP accumulation (Figures 2 and 3). Some of the androstenedione's effects may have been mediated by oestrogen. However, since dihydrotestosterone's effects were similar, it is suggestive that more than one class of follicular steroid can modify FSH stimulation of granulosa cell maturation; and that at least with regard to LH receptor induction, androgens do not appear to be atretogenic in porcine granulosa cell cultures. Effects of androgens on progesterone secretion were inconclusive in these experiments, however; neither dihydrotestosterone nor androstenedione prevented gonadotrophin-stimulated progesterone secretion.

From the information we have so far on granulosa cell maturation, it appears that FSH, via cAMP, initiates several cellular changes including LH receptor induction and transition from predominantly oestrogen to progesterone secretion. In turn, steroids produced in the follicle such as androgens and oestrogens can potentiate or inhibit some of these gonadotrophin-induced changes. Further modulation also apparently comes from peptides produced within the follicle. Whether a follicle properly matures to be capable of ovulation and luteinization or becomes atretic may be due to a balance between exposure to gonadotrophins and relative concentrations of intrafollicular steroids and peptide factors. This concept will be discussed below.

ROLE OF LOCAL FOLLICULAR FLUID CYBERNINS IN CONTROL OF GRANULOSA CELL MATURATION

The control of follicle development includes not only anterior pituitary hormones (principally LH and FSH) but also local factors (cybernins) generated in the ovary itself. As the mammalian follicle matures and enlarges under the influence of FSH during the follicular phase of the cycle an increase in the ability to secrete oestrogen can be observed. Since changes in follicular activity associated with final maturation occur only in the dominant follicle(s), whereas the other smaller follicles are arrested or become atretic, it is thought that local factors play a role in controlling follicular maturation. Recent work in this laboratory has investigated whether various cybernins in follicular fluid obtained from small, medium or large porcine follicles may function as regulators of *in vitro* 'luteinization' in cultures of porcine granulosa cells (see reference 26 for review).

Granulosa cells from small (1–2 mm) immature porcine follicles have been cultured for periods of 1, 4 and 6 days in the presence of FSH ($0.1 \mu g \, ml^{-1}$), insulin (I; $1 \, mIU \, ml^{-1}$), cortisol (F; $0.01 \mu g \, ml^{-1}$), and thyroxine (T; $10^{-7} \, mol \, l^{-1}$) which induces functional LH/hCG receptors *in vitro* in an analogous manner to the acquisition of LH/hCG receptors observed with *in vivo* follicular maturation (Figure 5). Granulosa cells obtained from immature follicles and cultured in this fashion exhibit increased secretion of progesterone associated with increased specific binding of [^{125}I]hCG. In order to examine the role of intraovarian regulators in modulation of LH/hCG receptor induction, follicular fluid from either small (1–2 mm) or large (6–12 mm) porcine follicles was added to cultures of granulosa cells in addition to FSH + IFT. LH/hCG receptors were measured by specific [^{125}I]hCG binding, cell number was estimated by determination of culture DNA content and progesterone secretion was determined by radioimmunoassay. Fluid from small follicles inhibited both induction of LH/hCG

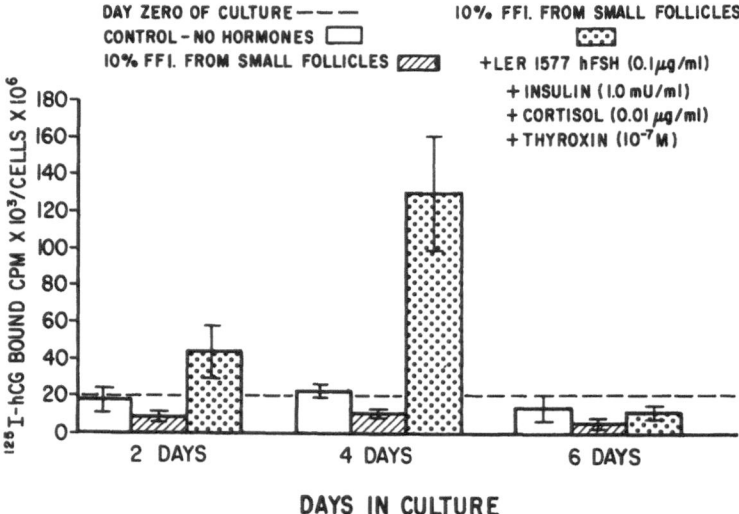

Figure 5 Effect of FSH plus insulin, cortisol and thyroxine upon the ability of porcine granulosa cells to bind iodinated hCG. Granulosa cells from small antral follicles of the pig were cultured for 2, 4 and 6 days in medium 199 and 10% pig serum containing either no exogenous hormones (control), hFSH (LER 8/117; 0.1 µg ml⁻¹), or hFSH (LER 8/117; 0.1 µg ml⁻¹) + insulin (1 mU ml⁻¹), cortisol (0.01 µg ml⁻¹) and thyroxine (10⁻⁷ mol l⁻¹). At the end of each incubation time the cells were removed from the flasks by scraping with a rubber policeman. Aliquots were removed for determination of specific binding of [¹²⁵I]hCG and DNA content of the cultured cells. The values represent the mean $\pm$ SE ($n = 4$) of two individual experiments. Day 0 represents the amount of [¹²⁵I]hCG bound to the cells on the day of collection

receptors (Figure 6) and progesterone section (Figure 7) when added at either 50%, 25%, or 12.5% to the cultures. In contrast to the inhibitory effects observed when fluid was added from small follicles, fluid from large, mature follicles was only slightly inhibitory of LH/hCG receptor induction (60–80% of maximum receptor induction can be observed with fluid from large follicles compared with only 25–50% observed with fluid from small follicles) and consistently stimulatory of progesterone secretion when 50% fluid was added to the cultures. Fluid from medium-sized follicles (not shown) has intermediate effects on both LH/hCG receptor induction and progesterone secretion compared with fluid from large and small follicles.

In preliminary studies in which the follicular fluids were subjected to Amicon PM-10 membrane filtration, we observed that the inhibitory activity of receptor induction by FSH resided both in < 10 000 and > 10 000 dalton fractions, the > 10 000 dalton fraction having the greater activity (Figure 8). A roughly comparable inhibitory influence was obtained upon FSH induction of progesterone secretion (Figure 9). Further studies in which the granulosa cell maturation inhibitor is further purified are being carried out. Ledwitz-Rigby and her colleagues have also identified inhibitory activity upon granulosa cell luteinization in porcine follicular fluid obtained from small antral follicles which is absent in fluid obtained from large preovulatory follicles[27,28]. The inhibitory activity inhibits both morphological luteinization and LH stimulatable cyclic AMP accumulation[29,30]. Ledwitz-Rigby and Rigby[31] and Stewart et al.[28] further demonstrated

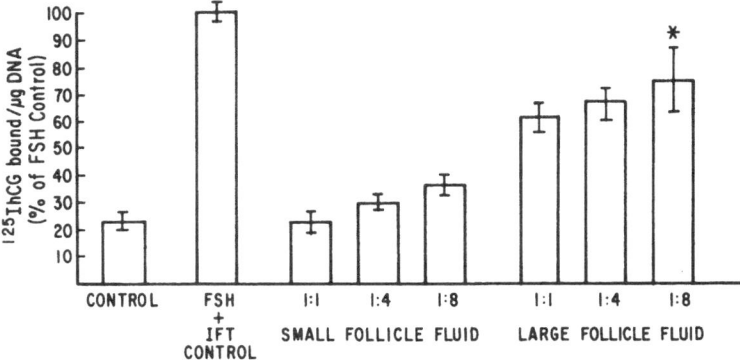

Figure 6 Effect of various doses of follicular fluid obtained from small (left) or large (right) porcine follicles upon FSH stimulation of LH/hCG receptors in cultured porcine granulosa cells. Granulosa cells from small antral porcine follicles were cultured for 4 days in 0.5 ml TC Media 199 and 10% pig serum containing either no exogenous hormone (control), FSH-IFT (hFSH, 0.1 µg ml^{-1} LER 8/117, 1 mU ml^{-1} insulin, 0.01 µg ml^{-1} hydrocortisone, 10^{-7} mol l^{-1} thyroxine) or FSH + IFT with 50, 25 or 12.5% whole porcine follicular fluid replacing part of the culture media. At the end of the culture period, cells were removed from the wells by scraping with a rubber policeman in physiological saline. Aliquots of the cells were taken for determination of [^{125}I]hCG binding and for DNA content. The values represent the mean $\pm$ SE for three separate experiments ($n = 6$). All of the cultures except the 'control' (far left) contained FSH-IFT (Taken from reference 26, with permission.)

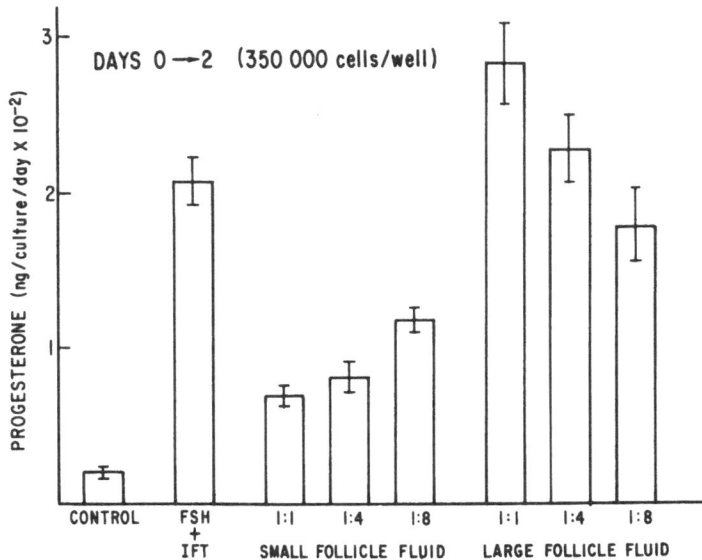

Figure 7 Effect of follicular fluid from small (left) and large (right) porcine follicles upon FSH stimulation of progesterone secretion by cultured porcine granulosa cells. Granulosa cells from small antral porcine follicles were cultured for 4 days in 0.5 ml TC Media 199 and 10% pig serum containing either no exogenous hormone (control), FSH-IFT (hFSH; LER 8/117; 0.1 µg ml^{-1}, 1 mU ml^{-1} insulin, 0.01 µg ml^{-1} hydrocortisone, 10^{-7} mol l^{-1} thyroxine) or FSH + IFT with 50, 25 or 12.5% whole porcine follicular fluid replacing part of the culture media. After 2 days of culture, media was changed and the 'spent' media assessed for progesterone content by specific radioimmunoassay. The values represent the mean $\pm$ SE for three separate experiments ($n = 12$). It should be noted that FSH + IFT was present in all the cultures except the 'control' (far left) (Taken from reference 26, with permission.)

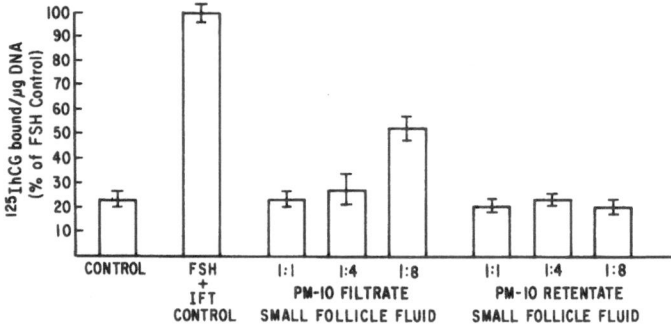

Figure 8 Effect of low (PM-10 filtrate, left) and high molecular weight (PM-10 retentate, right) fractions of follicular fluid obtained from small porcine follicles upon FSH stimulation of hCG/LH receptors in porcine granulosa cell cultures. Granulosa cells from small antral porcine follicles were cultured for 4 days in 0.5 ml TC Media 199 and 10% pig serum containing either no exogenous hormone (control), FSH-IFT (hFSH; LER 8/117; $0.1 \mu g \, ml^{-1}$, $1 \, mU \, ml^{-1}$ insulin, $0.01 \, \mu g \, ml^{-1}$ hydrocortisone, $10^{-7} \, mol \, l^{-1}$ thyroxine) or FSH + IFT with 50, 25 or 12.5% PM-10 filtrate ($< 10\,000$ daltons) or retentate ($> 10\,000$ daltons) of whole follicular fluid from small porcine follicles replacing part of the culture media. At the end of the culture period, cells were removed from the wells by scraping with a rubber policeman in physiological saline. Aliquots of the cells were taken for determination of $[^{125}I]hCG$ binding and for DNA content. The values represent the mean $\pm$ SE for three separate experiments ($n = 6$). It should be noted that all of the cultures except the 'control' (far left) contained FSH-IFT (Taken from reference 26, with permission.)

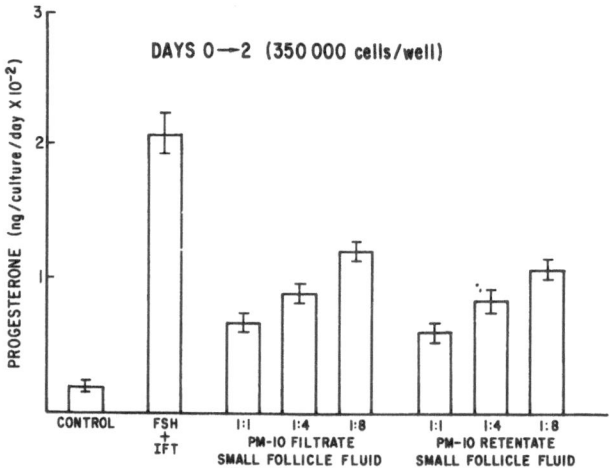

Figure 9 Effect of low (PM-10 filtrate, left) and high (PM-10 retentate, right) molecular weight fractions of follicular fluid upon FSH stimulation of progesterone secretion by cultured porcine granulosa cells. Granulosa cells from small antral porcine follicles were cultured for 4 days in 0.5 ml TC Media 199 and 10% pig serum containing either no exogenous hormone (control), FSH-IFT (hFSH; LER 8/117; $0.1 \mu g \, ml^{-1}$ insulin, $0.01 \, \mu g \, ml^{-1}$ hydrocortisone, $10^{-7} \, mol \, l^{-1}$ thyroxine) or FSH-IFT with 50, 25 or 12.5% PM-10 filtrate ($< 10\,000$ daltons) or retentate ($> 10\,000$ daltons) of whole follicular fluid from small porcine follicles replacing part of the culture media. After 2 days of culture, media was changed and the 'spent' media assessed for progesterone content by specific radioimmunoassay. The values represent the mean $\pm$ SE for three separate experiments ($n = 12$). It should be noted that FSH-IFT was present in all of the cultures except the 'control' (far left) (Taken from reference 26, with permission.)

a luteinization stimulator in fluid from large porcine follicles which enhances LH and FSH stimulation of progesterone secretion in porcine granulosa cell cultures. Kolena and Channing have also found that the stimulatory fraction in fluid from large preovulatory pig follicles enhances FSH induction of LH receptors[26] in addition to stimulating progesterone secretion. Kolena and Channing obtained a 32-fold purification of the stimulator using gel filtration chromatography on Sephadex G-100 and DEAE Sephacel ion exchange chromatography[32]. Further studies on purification are being carried out.

A balance between luteinization inhibitor and stimulators probably enables a follicle to mature, ovulate and luteinize rather than become atretic (Figure 10).

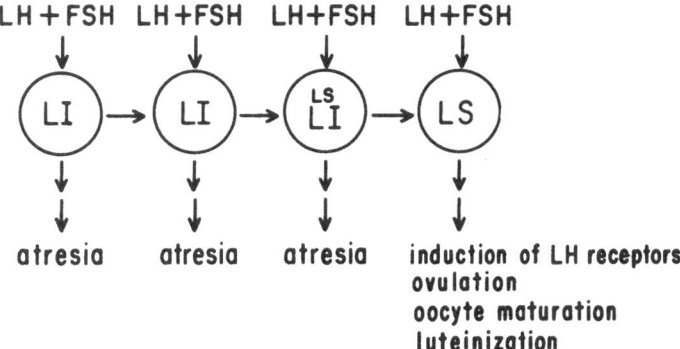

Figure 10 Diagrammatic representation of the proposed role for LI/LS in the maturational process of the ovarian follicle

GRANULOSA CELL SECRETION OF LOCAL CYBERNINS *IN VIVO*

The oocyte remains in the immature dictyate state of maturation until immediately prior to ovulation at which time it completes its maturation, including breakdown of the germinal vesicle and extrusion of the first polar body. This maturation process is essential to render the oocyte fertilizable. If an immature oocyte is removed from a medium-sized follicle and cultured it will mature spontaneously; if follicular fluid is added back to the cultured oocyte, maturation is arrested[33–36]. The inhibitor of oocyte maturation (OMI) in porcine follicular fluid has been partially purified by Tsafriri *et al.*[37], Stone *et al.*[36], Pomerantz *et al.*[38], Gwatkin and Anderson[39] and reviewed in Channing *et al.*[26]. The putative OMI is a polypeptide of < 2000 daltons, most likely < 1000 daltons. Granulosa cells, not thecal tissue, can secrete the OMI[34, 35]. Recent studies have shown that OMI is secreted in greater amounts by granulosa cells obtained from small immature follicles compared with granulosa cells obtained from large preovulatory follicles[26] (Figure 11). Addition of FSH and prolactin to cultured granulosa cells obtained from small and medium-sized porcine follicles enhances their secretion of OMI[40, 41]. Addition of LH to these granulosa cell cultures has no effect upon the secretion of OMI. In contrast, addition of testosterone $1.4 \mu g\,ml^{-1}$, but not oestradiol, led to a decrease in OMI secretion[40]. It is therefore possible that FSH enhances follicle viability by maintaining the ability of granulosa cells to secrete oestrogen and OMI. The preovulatory surge of LH could act on the follicle to eventually decrease OMI by bringing about granulosa cell luteinization and thus decrease their ability to secrete OMI. In addition the preovulatory surge of LH could act upon the theca interna to enhance thecal androgen secretion which could in turn act to decrease granulosa cell OMI secretion. Further studies are needed before these possibilities are adequately understood.

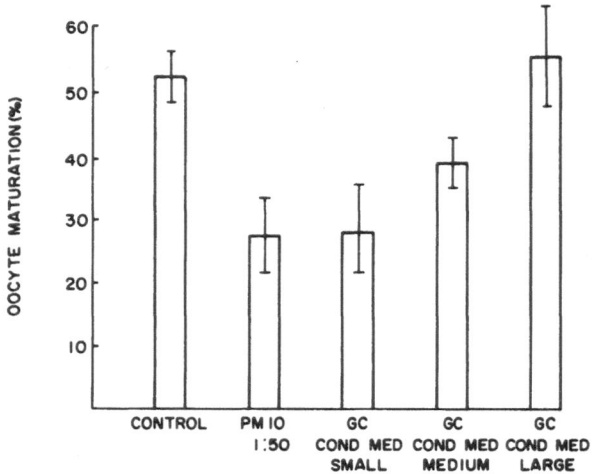

Figure 11 Inhibitory effect of conditioned porcine granulosa cell culture medium upon porcine oocyte maturation. Porcine granulosa cells from small (1–2 mm), medium (3–5 mm) and large follicles (6–12 mm) were cultured for 48 h and the conditioned medium filtered through Amicon PM-10 filters. The PM-10 filtrate was added to porcine oocytes (50–60/test) and the effect on oocyte maturation determined after 2 days of incubation in media consisting of one part conditioned medium and one part TC 199A. Data are expressed as mean ± SE of 6–8 experiments

Besides keeping the egg in the arrested state, low molecular weight components of porcine follicular fluid also inhibit progesterone secretion and outgrowth of cumulus cells from cultured cumulus-enclosed porcine oocytes[42]. Whether this inhibitory activity upon cumulus cells is due to the same compound as inhibition of nuclear maturation of oocytes cannot be determined until this material is purified to homogeneity. Interestingly, low molecular weight fractions of porcine follicular fluid also inhibited outgrowth (monolayer formation) as well as progesterone secretion by clumps of porcine granulosa cells[26]. When the low molecular weight fraction ($< 10\,000$ dalton Amicon PM-10 membrane filtration) of porcine follicular fluid is chromatographed on Sephadex G-25 the inhibitory activity upon oocyte maturation, granulosa cell clump outgrowth and granulosa cell progesterone secretion co-elute[26]. Subsequent chromatography on CM-Sephadex using a stepwise gradient of ammonium acetate (pH 5.5) separates the bulk of impurities from the OMI activity and clump outgrowth inhibitory activity; OMI activity elutes principally after $0.05\,\mathrm{mol\,l^{-1}}$ and $0.1\,\mathrm{mol\,l^{-1}}$ (late) ammonium acetate and clump outgrowth inhibitory activity elutes after both 0.05 and $0.1\,\mathrm{mol\,l^{-1}}$ (early) ammonium acetate steps. Further studies on purification of these two activities from follicular fluid will be required to resolve whether they are indeed two separate compounds or whether there is heterogeneity of one or both activities.

GRANULOSA CELL SECRETION OF LOCAL CYBERNINS *IN VITRO*

In order to see if porcine granulosa cells could secrete material *in vitro* capable of inhibiting granulosa cell outgrowth and oocyte maturation, granulosa cells were harvested from small and medium-sized porcine follicles and cultured for up to $2\frac{1}{2}$ days in tissue culture Medium 199 plus 10% pig serum. At the end of the incubation the conditioned media was subjected to purification procedures which included Amicon PM-10 membrane filtration, Sephadex G-10 column chromatography and CM-Sephadex chromatography using 0.01 mol l^{-1} ammonium acetate at pH 5.0. The ability of each fraction to inhibit outgrowth of cultured granulosa cell aggregates was assessed. The final product eluted from the CM-Sephadex column was also evaluated for ability to inhibit maturation of cultured porcine cumulus-enclosed oocytes. The activity which both inhibited oocyte maturation and outgrowth of granulosa cell aggregates behaves like a low molecular weight acidic material; it passes through the Amicon PM-10 membrane and elutes beyond the void volume of the G-10 column and is not retained on the CM-Sephadex column at pH 5. A stimulator of outgrowth of granulosa cell aggregates separates from the inhibitor on the Sephadex G-10 column, eluting prior to the inhibitor. No inhibitory or stimulatory activity is recovered from blank culture medium. It is concluded that porcine granulosa cells secrete low molecular weight material(s) which is capable of inhibiting outgrowth of granulosa and cumulus cells as well as oocyte maturation.

A summary of the purification of the granulosa cell monolayer formation inhibitor is shown in Table 1. About a 20-fold purification has been achieved. Granulosa cell aggregates incubated in the presence of the inhibitor remain rounded (Figure 12, bottom panel) whereas the aggregates form a monolayer

Table 1 Activity of porcine granulosa cell monolayer inhibitor

Sample	Absorbance (230 nm)	Peptide (mg ml^{-1})*	Units $(\text{mg peptide})^{-1}$†	Total units
PM-10 (concentrate)	35.75	59.84	0.21	151
G-10 I	3.02	20.86	0.64	280
G-10 II	1.14	5.87	0.83	90
CM-Sephadex	0.57	1.50	4.17	100

*Peptide was determined by fluorescamine assay.
†One unit inhibits monolayer formation by 50%.

Porcine granulosa cells were grown in 10^8 cell aliquots at a concentration of $10^6 \text{ cells ml}^{-1}$ in TC 199 + 10% porcine serum for 48 h followed by centrifugation, treatment of the medium for 30 min with 1 mmol l^{-1} PMSF and freezing of the conditioned medium. When 1 l of medium was accumulated it was pooled and subjected to PM-10 filtration and lyophilization of the PM-10 filtrate. The PM-10 filtrate was assayed at four doses in the granulosa cell clump monolayer assay using 100–200 granulosa cell clumps/dose. The PM-10 filtrate was chromatographed on Sephadex G-10 followed by rechromatography on Sephadex G-10 and finally by chromatography on CM-Sephadex.

under control culture conditions. The inhibitory effect upon monolayer formation is reversible[26]. When the PM-10 filtrate is chromatographed on Sephadex G-10 and the principal inhibitory material rechromatographed on Sephadex G-10 (Figure 13) the material is resolved into a stimulator fraction eluting early

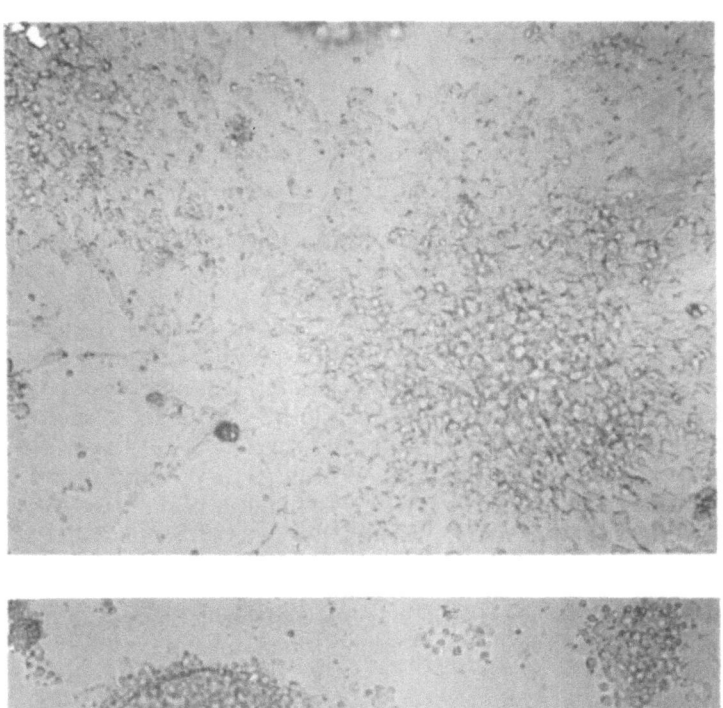

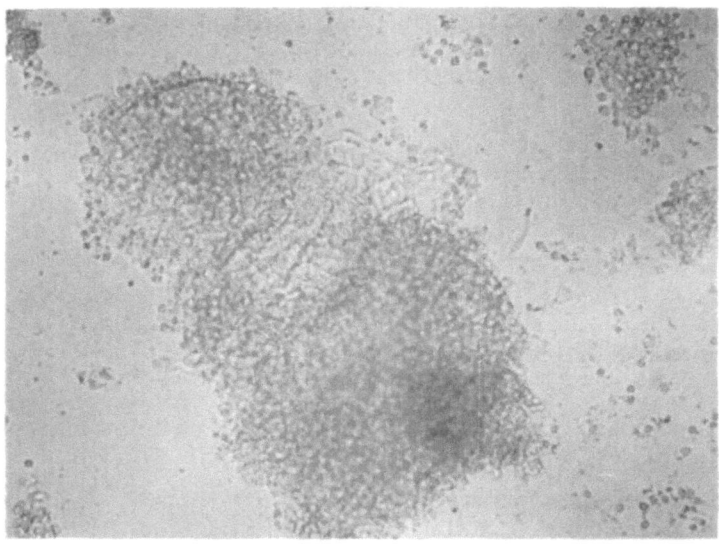

Figure 12 Appearance of clumps of porcine granulosa cells after culture for 24 h in the presence of control medium (top panel) and in the presence of $\frac{1}{50}$ dilution of low molecular weight concentrate of porcine follicular fluid (bottom panel). Note that the cells have formed a monolayer under control conditions (top) and that they remain clumped when they are cultured in the presence of the low molecular weight fraction of porcine follicular fluid (bottom)

(fractions 45–50) and an inhibitor eluting later (fractions 55–80). This is a consistent finding and was found in at least four batches of conditioned granulosa cell medium. This stimulator warrants further study. Interestingly, in follicular fluid there is a luteinization inhibitor and stimulator. Whether these small peptides represent precursors which aggregate in the follicular fluid is not known but presents an attractive hypothesis. The elution pattern of the inhibitor using ion exchange chromatography on CM-Sephadex is shown in Figure 14. A dose–response effect of the inhibitor upon granulosa cell progesterone secretion and monolayer formation is shown in Table 2.

Table 2 Effect of partially purified stimulator and inhibitor recovered from conditioned porcine granulosa cell media upon granulosa aggregate monolayer formation and progesterone secretion by cultured granulosa cells

Treatment	Granulosa monolayer formation (%)	Progesterone secretion (ng ml^{-1} 24 h^{-1})
Control	35.0 (0.8)	10.2 (1.4)
Stimulator (G-10 II)	48.7 (5.6)*	13.4 (1.2)
Inhibitor (CM-Sephadex)		
full strength	0.7 (0.6)*	< 4.0
½ strength	9.9 (2.7)*	5.2 (0.8)*
¼ strength	28.5 (4.6)	4.4 (0.2)*
⅛ strength	40.7 (3.5)	7.9 (1.7)

*Significantly different from control value ($p \leqslant 0.025$).

Results are presented as mean $\pm$ SE. Each sample was added to four cultures of granulosa cells and the cultures incubated for 48 h. Granulosa cell monolayer formation was estimated after 24 h of culture and progesterone secretion in the culture was estimated after 48 h of culture.

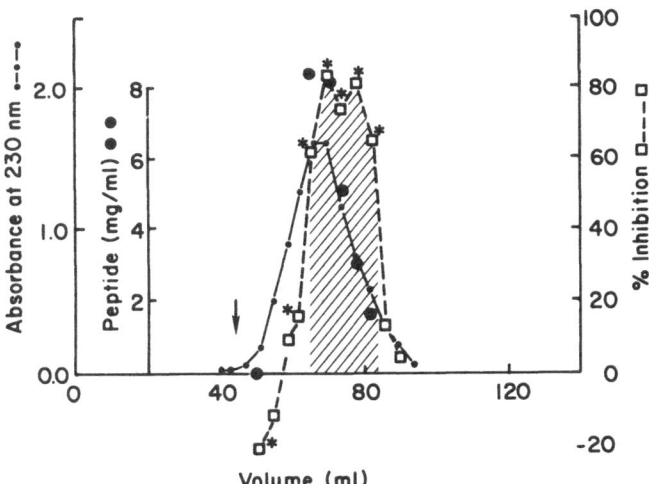

Figure 13 Re-chromatography of inhibitory fractions from first Sephadex column on Sephadex G-10; 10 ml, containing 26.3 mg peptide ml^{-1}, were applied to the 2.5 × 25 cm column and eluted with distilled water—4 ml fractions were collected. Samples were diluted four times for granulosa monolayer assay. Results are presented as mean percentage inhibition of monolayer formation. Asterisks indicate fractions which significantly inhibited monolayer formation ($p < 0.001$) using χ^2 analysis. The void volume is indicated by the arrow. The peptide content of individual fractions was determined by fluorescamine method; note that a stimulatory material eluted before the inhibitory material

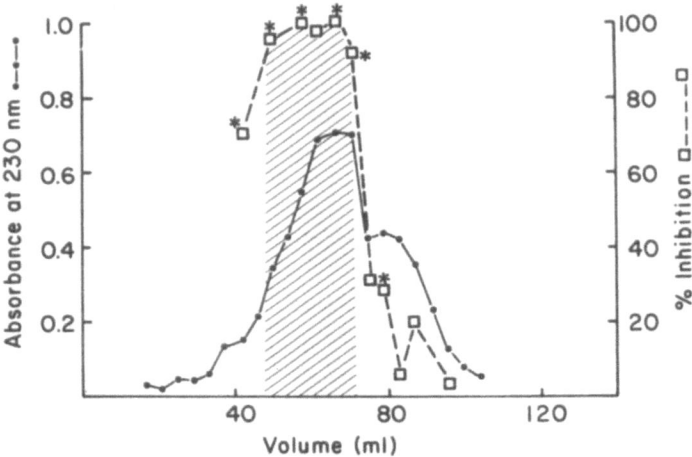

Figure 14 Ion exchange chromatography of Sephadex G-10 II purified inhibitory material on CM-Sephadex. A 17.5 ml sample containing 5.87 mg peptide ml^{-1} was applied to the 2×25 cm column. Elution was accomplished with the starting buffer, 0.01 mol l^{-1} ammonium acetate, pH 5.0; 4 ml fractions were collected. Aliquots were diluted 2.2 times for monolayer assay. Asterisks indicate those fractions which significantly inhibited monolayer formation ($p < 0.02$). Fractions indicated by shaded area in Figure 13 were pooled to form the CM-Sephadex sample

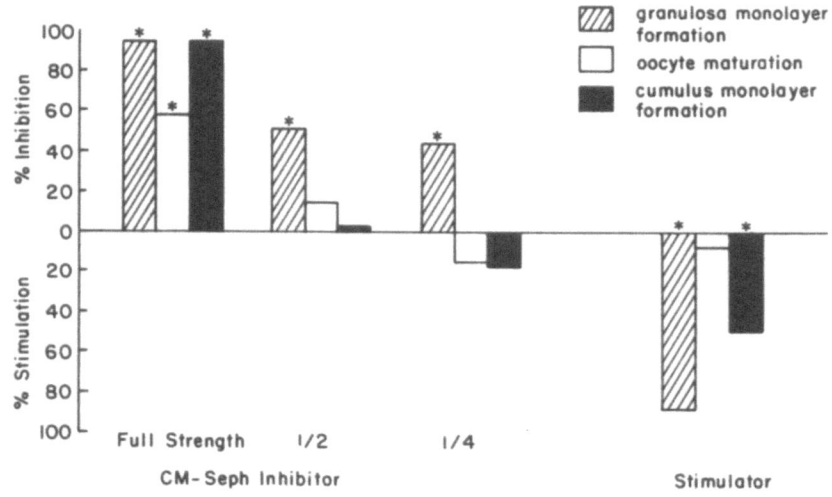

Figure 15 Comparison of the effects of granulosa monolayer inhibitor purified by CM-Sephadex chromatography and stimulator purified by Sephadex G-10 chromatography on granulosa mono-layer formation, oocyte maturation and cumulus cell monolayer formation by cultured porcine cumulus enclosed oocytes and granulosa cell clumps. The final concentration of the inhibitor was 0.6 mg peptide ml^{-1} at full strength. Final concentration of the stimulator was 29.3 µg peptide ml^{-1}. The asterisks indicate those values significantly different from the control ($p < 0.001$). The cumulus-enclosed oocytes were cultured for 48 h and progesterone measured in the conditioned culture medium[42] and nuclear maturation evaluated in the oocytes as detailed by Tsafriri and Channing[34,35]

The stimulator significantly enhances monolayer formation by cultured granulosa cells whereas the inhibitor leads to a dose dependent inhibition of granulosa cell outgrowth and progesterone secretion. When the effects of the inhibitor and stimulator are examined upon oocyte maturation it is evident that the inhibitor produces a dose dependent inhibition of both oocyte maturation and cumulus cell outgrowth as well as granulosa cell outgrowth (Figure 15). The stimulator enhances both cumulus and granulosa cell outgrowth but has no effect upon oocyte maturation. This is most likely because oocyte maturation in culture is already 'maximal' and cannot be stimulated further. A stimulator of oocyte maturation could also exist in follicular fluid. Indirect evidence for this exists in our purification procedures of OMI from porcine follicular fluid in which we have observed a greater than 100% recovery of OMI activity in CM-Sephadex fractions compared with the starting PM-10 filtrate of porcine follicular fluid[26]. This finding could be explained by separation of the stimulator from the inhibitor. Studies in which the stimulator is mixed with the inhibitor originating from follicular fluid and conditioned granulosa cell medium will be carried out in order to see if they each can neutralize the activity of the other on oocytes.

In conclusion, the follicular events of maturation which lead to ovulation and luteinization of the follicle appear to be directed not only by gonadotrophins but also by intrafollicular substances, both steroidal and non-steroidal, which may act alone and/or modulate gonadotrophin-mediated effects on the various maturational events.

Acknowledgements

Supported in part by grants from the National Institute of Child Health and Human Development HDO8834 and the Ford Foundation 7600530A.

References

1. Channing, C. P., Thanki, K. H., Lindsey, A. and Ledwitz-Rigby, F. (1978). Development and hormonal regulation of gonadotropin responsiveness in granulosa cells of the mammalian ovary. In *Receptors and Hormone Action*. Vol. III. (New York: Academic Press)
2. Hillier, S. G. (1981). Regulation of follicular oestrogen biosynthesis: A summary of current concepts. *J. Endocrinol.*, **89**, 3P
3. Zeleznik, A. J., Midgley, A. R. and Reichert, L. E. (1974). Granulosa cell maturation in the rat: Increased binding of human chorionic gonadotropin following treatment with follicle-stimulating hormone *in vivo*. *Endocrinology*, **95**, 818
4. Channing, C. P. (1975). Follicle stimulating hormone stimulation of ^{125}I-human chorionic gonadotropin binding in porcine granulosa cell cultures. *Proc. Soc. Exp. Biol. Med.*, **149**, 238
5. May, J. V., McCathy, K., Reichert, L. E. and Schomberg, D. W. (1980). Follicle stimulating hormone-mediated induction of functional luteinizing hormone/human chorionic gonadotropin receptors during monolayer culture of porcine granulosa cells. *Endocrinology*, **107**, 1041
6. Thanki, K. H. and Channing, C. P. (1976). Influence of serum, estrogen and gonadotropins upon growth and progesterone secretion by cultures of granulosa cells from small porcine follicles. *Endocr. Res. Commun.*, **3**, 319
7. Schaerf, F. W., Anderson, L. D. and Channing, C. P. (1984). Steroidogenesis by porcine granulosa cells: Temporal pattern of estrogen and progesterone secretion *in vitro*. (In press)
8. Rayford, P. L., Brinkley, H. J., Young, E. P. and Reichert, L. E. (1974). Radioimmunoassay of porcine FSH. *J. Anim. Sci.*, **39**, 348
9. Niswender, G. D., Reichert, L. E. and Zimmerman, D. R. (1970). Radioimmunoassay of serum levels of luteinizing hormone throughout the estrous cycle in pigs. *Endocrinology*, **87**, 576
10. Channing, C. P. and Kammerman, S. (1973). Characteristics of gonadotropin receptors of porcine granulosa cells during follicle maturation. *Endocrinology*, **92**, 531
11. Lindsey, A. M. and Channing, C. P. (1979). Influence of follicular maturation upon cyclic AMP accumulation by isolated porcine granulosa cells. *Biol. Reprod.*, **20**, 473

12. Kammerman, S. and Ross, J. (1975). Increase in numbers of gonadotropin receptors on granulosa cells during follicle maturation. *J. Clin. Endocrinol. Metab.*, **41**, 546
13. Loeken, M. L. and Channing, C. P. (1981). Induction of functional receptors for luteinizing hormone by follicle stimulating hormone and estradiol 17-β in cultured porcine granulosa cells. *Biol. Reprod. Suppl.*, **24**, 123
14. Loeken, M. (1982). Follicle stimulating hormone requires protein synthesis to cause granulosa cell maturation. *Endocrinol. Suppl.*, **110**, 760
15. Loeken, M. L. and Channing, C. P. (1984). Interaction of estradiol 17-β with follicle stimulating hormone on induction of functional receptors for luteinizing hormone in cultured porcine granulosa cells. (In press)
16. Richards, J. S., Ireland, J. J., Rao, M. C., Bernath, G. A., Midgley, A. R. and Reichert, L. E. (1976). Ovarian follicular development in the rat: Hormone receptor regulation by estradiol, follicle stimulating hormone and luteinizing hormone. *Endocrinology*, **99**, 1562
17. Stouffer, R. L., Nixon, W. E. and Hodgen, G. D. (1977). Estrogen inhibition of basal and gonadotropin-stimulated progesterone production by rhesus monkey luteal cells *in vitro*. *Endocrinology*, **101**, 1157
18. Haney, A. F. and Schomberg, D. W. (1978). Steroidal modulation of progesterone secretion by granulosa cells from large porcine follicles: A role for androgens and estrogens in controlling steroidogenesis. *Biol. Reprod.*, **19**, 242
19. Williams, M. T. and Marsh, J. M. (1978). Estradiol inhibition of luteinizing hormone-stimulated progesterone synthesis in isolated bovine luteal cells. *Endocrinology*, **103**, 1611
20. Fortune, J. E. and Hansel, W. (1979). The effects of 17β–estradiol on progesterone secretion by bovine theca and granulosa cells. *Endocrinology*, **104**, 1834
21. Rani, S. S., Salhanick, A. R. and Armstrong, D. T. (1981). Follicle-stimulating hormone induction of luteinizing hormone receptor in cultured rat granulosa cells: An examination of the need for steroids in the induction process. *Endocrinology*, **108**, 1379
22. Veldhuis, J. D., Klase, P. A. and Hammond, J. M. (1981). Direct actions of 17β-estradiol on progesterone production by highly differentiated porcine granulosa cells *in vitro*. II. Regulatory interactions of estradiol with luteinizing hormone and cyclic nucleotides. *Endocrinology*, **109**, 433
23. McNatty, K. P., Moore-Smith, D., Osathanondh, R. and Ryan, K. J. (1979). The human antral follicle: Functional correlates of growth and atresia. *Ann. Biol. Anim. Bioch. Biophys.*, **19**, 1547
24. Farookhi, R. (1980). Effects of androgen on induction of gonadotropin receptors and gonadotropin-stimulated adenosine 3′, 5′–monophosphate production in rat ovarian granulosa cells. *Endocrinology*, **106**, 1216
25. Nimrod, A. (1981). On the synergestic action of androgen and FSH on progestin secretion by cultured rat granulosa cells. *Mol. Cell. Endocrinol.*, **21**, 51
26. Channing, C. P., Anderson, L. D., Hoover, D. J., *et al.* (1982). The role of non-steroidal regulators in control of oocyte and follicular maturation. *Rec. Prog. Horm. Res.*, **38**, 331
27. Ledwitz-Rigby, F., Rigby, B. W., Gay, V. L., Stetson, M., Young, J. and Channing, C. P. (1977). Inhibitory action of porcine follicular fluid upon granulosa cell luteinization *in vitro*: Assay and influence of follicular maturation. *J. Endocrinol.*, **74**, 175
28. Stewart, L. E., Rigby, B. W. and Ledwitz-Rigby, F. (1982). Follicular fluid stimulation of progesterone secretion time course, dose response and effect of inhibiting *de novo* cholesterol synthesis. *Biol. Reprod.*, **27**, 54
29. Ledwitz-Rigby, F. (1980). Reversal of follicular fluid inhibition of granulosa cell progesterone secretion by manipulation of intracellular cyclic AMP. *Biol. Reprod.*, **23**, 324
30. Ledwitz-Rigby, F. and Rigby, B. W. (1981). Ovarian inhibitors and stimulators of granulosa cell maturation and luteinization. In Franchimont, P. and Channing, C. P. (eds.) *Intragonadal Regulation of Reproduction.* pp. 97–131. (New York: Academic Press)
31. Ledwitz-Rigby, F. and Rigby, B. (1979). Follicular fluid stimulation of steroidogenesis in immature granulosa cells *in vitro*. *Mol. Cell. Endocrinol.*, **14**, 73
32. Kolena, J. and Channing, C. P. (1984). Stimulatory action of follicular fluid components on maturation of granulosa cells from small porcine follicles. (In press)
33. Chang, M. C. (1955). The maturation of rabbit oocytes in culture and their maturation, activation, fertilization and subsequent development in the fallopian tubes. *J. Exp. Zool.*, **128**, 379
34. Tsafriri, A. and Channing, C. P. (1975a). An inhibitory influence of granulosa cells and follicular fluid upon porcine oocyte meiosis *in vitro*. *Endocrinology*, **96**, 922
35. Tsafriri, A. and Channing, C. P. (1975b). Influence of follicular maturation and culture conditions on the meiosis of pig oocytes *in vitro*. *J. Reprod. Fertil.*, **43**, 149

36. Stone, S. L., Pomerantz, S. H., Schwartz-Kripner, A. and Channing, C. P. (1978). Inhibitor of oocyte maturation from porcine follicular fluid: Further purification and evidence for reversible action. *Biol. Reprod.*, **19**, 585

37. Tsafriri, A., Pomerantz, S. H. and Channing, C. P. (1976). Inhibition of oocyte maturation by porcine follicular fluid: Partial characterization of the inhibitor. *Biol. Reprod.*, **14**, 511

38. Pomerantz, S. H., Channing, C. P. and Tsafriri, A. (1979). Studies on the purification and action of an oocyte maturation inhibitor isolated from porcine follicular fluid. In Gross, E. and Meinhofer, J. (eds.) *Peptides: Structure and Biological Function*, pp. 765–74. (Pierce Chemical Co.)

39. Gwatkin, R. B. L. and Anderson, O. F. (1976). Hamster oocyte maturation *in vitro*: Inhibition by follicular components. *Life Sci.*, **19**, 527

40. Anderson, L., Stone, S. L. and Channing, C. P. (1980). Hormonal control of oocyte maturation (OMI) secretion from porcine granulosa cells. Abstract 358. *Presented at the 62nd Annual Meeting of the Endocrine Society*, June 18–20, Washington D.C.

41. Channing, C. P. and Evans, V. (1982). Stimulatory effect of ovine prolactin upon cultured porcine granulosa cell secretion of inhibitory activity of oocyte maturation. *Endocrinology*, **111**, 1746

42. Hillensjö, T., Pomerantz, S. H., Schwartz-Kripner, A., Anderson, L. D. and Channing, C. P. (1980). Inhibition of cumulus cell progesterone secretion by low molecular weight fractions of porcine follicular fluid which also inhibit oocyte maturation. *Endocrinology*, **106**, 584

43. Nakano, R., Akahori, T., Katayama, K. and Tojo, S. (1977). Binding of LH and FSH to porcine granulosa cells during follicle maturation. *J. Reprod. Fertil.*, **51**, 23

44. Lanning, C. P., Schaerf, F. W., Anderson, L. D. and Tsafriri, A. (1980). Ovarian follicular and luteal physiology. *Int. Rev. Physiol.*, **22**, 117

5
Influence of cyclic variations in gonadotrophin and steroid hormones on follicular growth in the human ovary

A. Gougeon

INTRODUCTION

During the menstrual cycle both endocrine and morphological changes affect the ovarian follicle population. Except for the final preovulatory phase of follicular maturation[1] little is known of the morphological changes affecting the various categories of follicles throughout the cycle in spite of the elegant studies of Koering[2] in the macaque, and Block[3] in the human. The efforts of these last two authors revealed several features of folliculogenesis in primates, their studies having described cyclic variations in the size of follicles and the level of atresia.

In the human species, the data established by Block[3] primarily concerned follicles of over 1 mm diameter. It is therefore impossible from these results alone to determine the controlling influences upon all the different stages of follicular development from the differentiation of the theca interna (diameter about 150 μm) right up to ovulation (about 20 000 μm diameter).

The aim of this study was to analyse the morphometric changes of those follicles possessing a theca interna throughout the cycle. These follicles were classified into eight categories. Differences in follicle diameter, class size, mitotic index and follicle quality were considered in relation to cyclic changes in gonadotrophins and steroids according to accepted published figures[4-7].

MATERIALS AND METHODS

Sampling

Fifty ovaries and six large ovarian wedge resections were obtained from 33 women during gynaecological surgery (ovariectomy for carcinoma of the breast or cervix, hysterectomy for fibroids). The ages of the patients varied between 18 and 50 years.

The ovaries were fixed in either Bouin's fluid or a mixture of alcohol, formaldehyde and acetic acid, processed by routine histological methods and then serially sectioned at 10 μm.

Ovarian function was considered to be normal after verification of the following criteria:

(1) Absence of morphological pathology of the ovary.
(2) Regular cycles: 28 ± 2 days (determined over the previous three cycles).
(3) In hysterectomy cases the histological appearance of the endometrium had to agree with the stage of the cycle when surgery was performed.
(4) Peripheral levels of LH, FSH, oestradiol and progesterone were determined by radioimmunoassay in 12 women. These values all had to be within the ranges described for normal women[4,5].
(5) Ovulation had to have occurred in each of the preceding three cycles, and be corroborated by the presence of cyclical corpora lutea at various stages of degeneration.

Determination of the menstrual cycle day

A theoretical 28-day menstrual cycle was used as reference, and divided into six stages of equal duration: early (days 1–5), mid- (days 6–10) and late (day 11 to ovulation) follicular phase, and early (days 15–19), mid- (days 20–24) and late (days 25–28) luteal phase.

The samples included in the study were classified into these cycle stages according to the dates of the last menstrual periods and the ovarian histology. For this last criterion, the stage of development of the preovulatory follicle[1] and the age of the cyclical corpus luteum[8] enabled the samples to be dated with good precision.

Classification of follicles

The 2125 follicles showing a theca interna were studied, since it is only upon acquisition of a theca interna (between 115 and 140 μm diameter) that the human follicle comes within the morphological scheme.

The gonadotrophin receptor content has not been determined in human preantral follicles. However, in the rat, Zeleznik et al.[9] have shown the presence of LH receptors in the theca interna from differentiation onwards, with FSH receptors appearing with the development of the granulosa[10]. One may therefore propose that in women as in the rat, the appearance of the theca interna coincides with a sensitization of the follicle to gonadotrophins.

These gonadotrophin-sensitive follicles were divided into eight groups according to the number of granulosa cells they contained (Figure 1).

Morphological parameters of follicular growth

These parameters reflecting the differential developmental capacity of the follicles in each class were determined for each of the classes 1 to 6 of granulosa cell content for the six stages of the theoretical 28-day cycle. The healthy follicles in classes 7 and 8 (usually only one per woman, and then only present durng the mid- and late follicular phases respectively) were not included in this analysis. Five parameters were determined, as shown in Table 1:

(1) The mean mitotic index of the healthy follicles, reflecting the growth rate of the follicles.

(2) The mean number of granulosa cells per healthy follicle, reflecting follicular size. The development of this parameter indicated the extent of movement of follicles from one class to the next. When the mean size of the follicles in a class diminishes, it indicates that there has been either an influx of follicles (whose granulosa cell number is at the lower limit for that class) into the class from the preceding class, or else the efflux of follicles (whose granulosa cell number is at the upper limit for the class) into the next class.

(3) The percentage of healthy follicles, this value being greater when there are fewer atretic follicles in the group. The development of this parameter is a good indicator of the cyclical effect on follicle atresia.

(4) The number of healthy + atretic follicles.

(5) The number of healthy follicles.

These last two parameters are expressed as a percentage of the total follicle population of all the classes combined. They need not necessarily vary in the same direction.

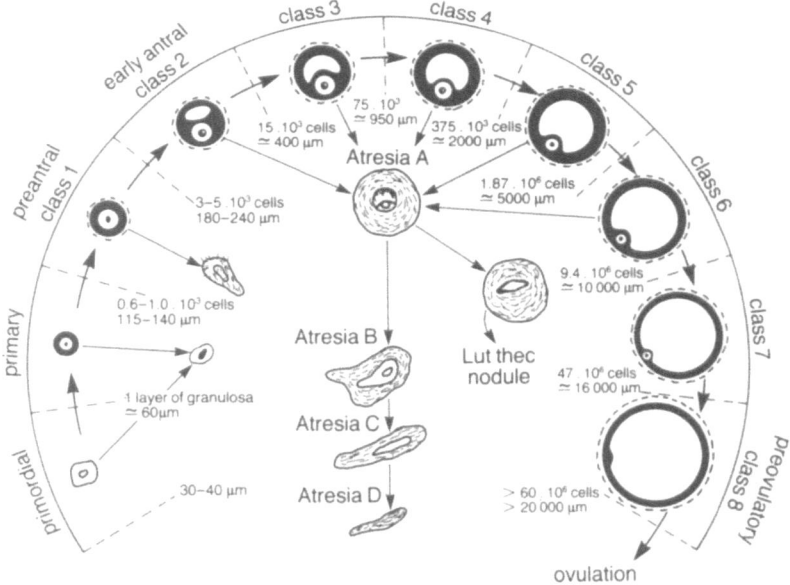

Figure 1 Classification of follicles within the human ovary. Adapted from Peters *et al.* (1978). *Clin. Endocrin. Metab.*, 7, 469; and Gougeon (1981). PhD Thesis, University of Paris

Statistical analysis

Analyses of variance and $\bar{\chi}^2$ tests were used to determine the significances of the observed changes.

RESULTS AND DISCUSSION

Variation in atresia during the cycle (Figure 2)

During the ovarian cycle, atresia affected the various classes of follicles differentially.

Table 1 Morphological parameters of follicular growth and their calculation

Mean mitotic index (per 10³ granulosa cells)

$$\overline{MI} = \frac{MI_1 + \ldots + MI_i + \ldots + MI_n}{n}$$

MI_i
- Number of mitoses in five sections ← Abercrombie's correction[10a] ← Number of mitoses seen in five sections
- Number of granulosa cells per mm³ (see G_i)
- Volume of granulosa corresponding to five sections { Follicle diameter (mm); Antrum diameter (mm); Oocyte diameter (mm)

Mean number of granulosa cells per healthy follicle

$$\overline{G} = \frac{G_1 + \ldots + G_i + \ldots + G_n}{n}$$

G_i
- Number of granulosa cells per mm³ ← Abercrombie's correction[10a] { Mean diameter of granulosa cell nuclei (mm); Section thickness; Number of granulosa cell nuclei per count area (graticule)
- Total volume of granulosa cells in follicle i (mm³) { Follicle diameter (mm); Mean depth of granulosa (4–100 estimations)

Percentage of healthy follicles

$$P = \frac{n_x \times 100}{N_x}$$

Number of healthy follicles

$$H = \frac{n_x \times 100}{N_1 + \ldots + N_8}$$

Number of healthy + atretic follicles

$$H + A = \frac{N_x \times 100}{N_1 + \ldots + N_8}$$

MI = Mitotic index; n = number of healthy follicles in class 'x'; N = number of healthy + atretic follicles in class 'x'; N_1 to N_8 = number of healthy + atretic follicles in classes 1 to 8; G = number of granulosa cells for a follicle i.

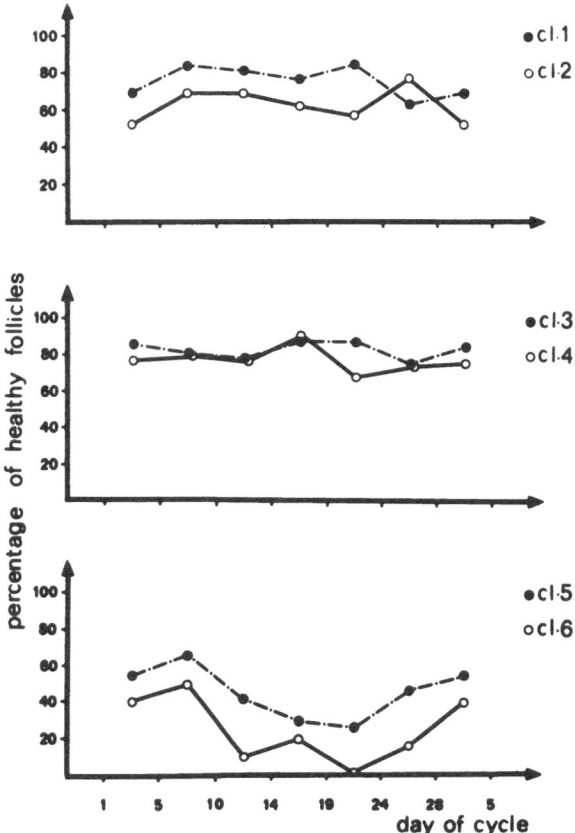

Figure 2 Variations in the percentages of healthy follicles in each class (cl.) during the ovarian cycle

The follicles in classes 1, 2, 3 and 4 (of about 140–2000 μm diameter) were only slightly affected by atresia. The mean percentages of healthy follicles in these classes were high, reaching 76 ± 3, 65 ± 3, 85 ± 3 and $76 \pm 3\%$, respectively. Furthermore, the variation in these percentages showed no cyclical pattern.

The behaviour of these follicles in classes 1–4 with respect to atresia is not peculiar to the human. In the cow, Choudary et al.[11] found no cyclical variation in the number of follicles of diameter under 5 mm, and the same has been reported for small antral follicles in the ewe[12].

Larger follicles of diameter over 2000 μm were highly susceptible to atresia. The mean percentages of healthy follicles in classes 5 and 6 were low, being only 42.0 ± 7 and $23 \pm 7\%$, respectively. In addition, there were large variations in these percentages within the cycle: atresia increased from the end of the follicular phase, remained high during the luteal phase and then declined at the end of the cycle.

This finding is contrary to the report of Block[3] who stated that for follicles of over 1 mm diameter while there was a decrease in atresia in the late follicular and mid-luteal phases, atresia was increased after ovulation and in the late luteal phase.

The present findings have allowed description of two fundamental character-istics of the influence exerted by the ovarian cycle upon the follicle population:

(1) The quality of the follicles in classes 1–4 is little influenced by the endocrine changes of the cycle.
(2) The quality of the follicles in classes 5 and 6 is highly dependent upon these endocrine changes. The higher the circulating levels of FSH (at the end and beginning of the ovarian cycle)[4,5] the higher the percentage of healthy follicles in these two classes. The role of FSH in regulating the number of large follicles (class 5 upwards) is therefore of prime importance in the human, just as it is in the rat[13,14], hamster[15], ewe[16] and, more generally, in all mammals[17].

Mitotic activity of granulosa cells in healthy follicles (Figure 3)

The mitotic activity of the follicles in classes 1, 3 and 4 showed no cyclical variation. However, that of the follicles in classes 2, 5 and 6 showed (sometimes highly) statistically significant variations.

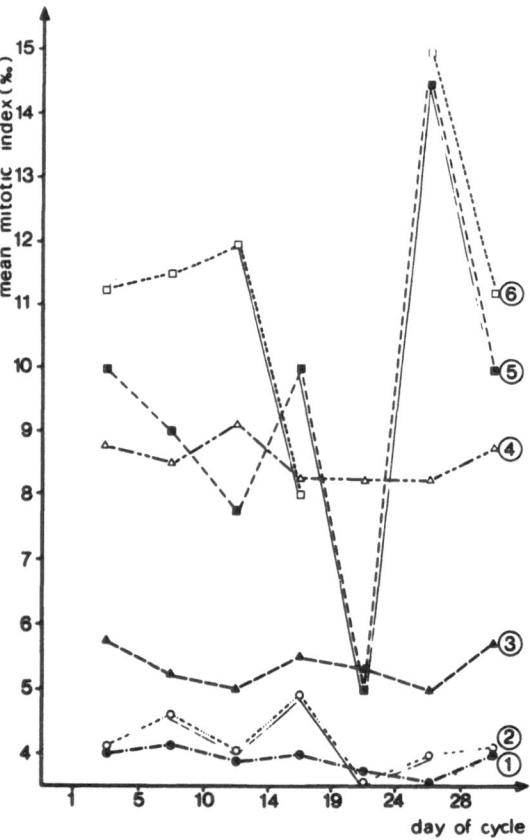

Figure 3 Variations in the mean mitotic activity of the granulosa for each class of follicles during the ovarian cycle. Statistically significant variations in the mitotic index are emphasized by a second solid line

Because the development of atresia in follicles belonging to classes 5 and 6 is directly dependent upon circulating FSH levels, and because this same hormone acts in the development of the antrum which characterizes class 2 follicles, classes 2, 5 and 6 appear to be the stages of follicular growth most sensitive to the action of FSH. It is therefore probable that the large variations in mitotic activity of these classes is related to their sensitivity to FSH. As these variations do not appear to be related to cyclic changes in this hormone, intraovarian factors may also be involved[18].

The only stage of the cycle where the mean mitotic index of the various classes showed an identical pattern of evolution was the mid-luteal phase (days 19–24). The follicles in classes 1, 3 and 4 had a low mitotic activity, and those in classes 2 and 5 had a very low mitotic activity. There was not a single healthy follicle found in class 6. The growth rate of all these follicles was clearly diminished.

It is in the mid-luteal phase that the secretory activity of the corpus luteum is maximal, synthesizing huge quantities of progesterone. The circulating levels of LH and FSH are very low at this time[4,5]. Progesterone is certainly responsible for this reduction in follicular activity as it lowers cell metabolism, slowing follicular growth (rat: Buffler and Roser[19]; rhesus monkey: Goodman and Hodgen[20]).

The mitotic activity of the granulosa of class 5 follicles was greatly elevated (from 5.00 ± 0.60 to $14.5 \pm 1.5\%$) in the late luteal phase. The mitotic index of the sole observed healthy follicle in class 6 was also greatly increased at 15.1%. This obvious increase in mitotic activity plays a leading role in the ensuing follicular growth. The follicle destined to ovulate in the following cycle comes from class 5 since it takes approximately 15 days for a follicle in this class to attain ovulatory size (class 8)[21].

At the end of the luteal phase the peripheral levels of progesterone fall dramatically, while gonadotrophin levels increase[4,5]. It is difficult to correlate this increase in follicular growth with either of these changes in the endocrine environment. Such an evolution is perhaps comparable with that described by Brand and de Jong[12] in the ewe where a wave of follicular development begins during the luteal phase, after the 14th day of the cycle, and with the fall in progesterone there is an acceleration in follicular growth up to ovulation.

Entry of follicles into classes 1 and 2 (Figure 4)

The results described below make it apparent that the simultaneous analysis of cyclical changes in certain morphological parameters of follicular growth is able to provide valuable information concerning the influence of the ovarian cycle as a regulator of follicular growth.

Entry of follicles into class 1 (Figure 4)

The only significant reduction during the cycle in the mean size of class 1 follicles was accompanied by a high percentage (76%) of healthy follicles in the class. It was also associated with an increase in the total number of follicles in the class. This reduction in the mean follicle size is therefore attributable to an entry of follicles into the class, and not an efflux into class 2.

This entry of follicles occurred at the start of the luteal phase (days 15–19), several days after the ovulatory discharge of gonadotrophins. Undoubtedly there is a direct relationship between the LH surge and the entry of follicles into class 1 since a small follicle enters class 1 when its theca interna differentiates under the control of LH[22].

Entry of follicles into class 2 (Figure 4)

The only significant fall in the mean size of class 2 follicles during the cycle was associated with a high percentage (69%) of healthy follicles in the class. It was also accompanied by a large and highly significant increase in the number of follicles in the class. Clearly this was attributable to an entry into the class of follicles from class 1, and not an efflux of follicles into class 3. This is confirmed by the simultaneous reduction of the number of class 1 follicles.

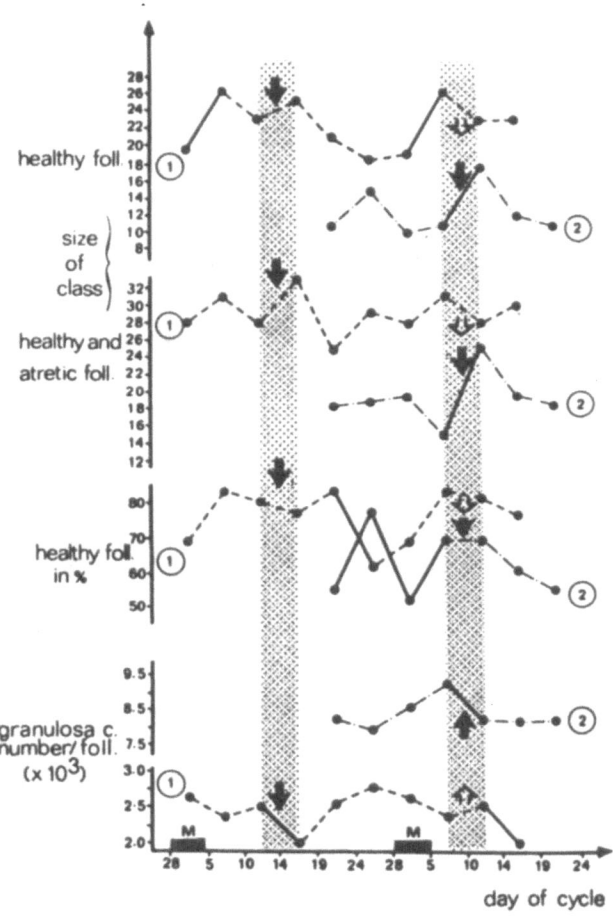

Figure 4 Development of four morphological parameters for classes 1 and 2 during the ovarian cycle. Statistically significant variations are denoted by unbroken lines. Solid arrows indicate the entry of follicles (foll.) into a class, and hollow arrows the efflux of follicles from one class into the next

It is in class 2 that the antrum develops. The entry of follicles into this class occurs in the late follicular phase (days 11–14). During this stage of the cycle the circulating levels of oestrogens, primarily originating from the preovulatory follicle[23], are appreciably elevated. If FSH is primarily responsible for the appearance of the antrum, then its action is greatly potentiated by these oestrogens[10].

This endocrine environment characterizing the late follicular phase is certainly responsible for the appearance of the antrum in a great number of the large preantral follicles and also induces the influx of follicles into class 2.

In conclusion, this study has shown that cyclical changes in the gonadotrophin and steroid hormone environment play two important roles in the regulation of follicular growth. Firstly, in controlling the number of large follicles (classes 5 and 6), which compete for selection culminating in the ovulation of a single follicle per cycle; and secondly, in favouring, at particular times in the cycle, the differentiation of the theca interna followed by the development of the antrum, and thereby inducing an influx of follicles into class 1 and 2. The time spent by follicles in class 1, i.e. the interval between the differentiation of the theca interna (entry into class 1) and the appearance of the antrum (entry into class 2), is 25 days[21]. It is therefore the same follicles which enter class 1 between days 15 and 19 of one cycle and enter class 2 between days 11 and 14 of the next.

Peters[24] and Richards[25] have suggested that the development of a follicle either to further growth stages or to atresia is dependent upon the time of the cycle being more or less favourable when that follicle developed its theca interna. The cyclic endocrine changes therefore initiate a wave of follicle growth whose first stages (classes 1 and 2) are exposed to high concentrations of LH, FSH and oestradiol-17β. These follicles will therefore be more resistant to atresia than those follicles having differentiated their theca interna and antra at other stages of the cycle under the less favourable influence of tonic secretory levels of gonadotrophins and steroids. It is from this wave of follicular development that the preovulatory follicle will come.

Acknowledgements

This work was supported by a grant from the Université Paris-Sud, UER Médicale Kremlin-Bicêtre (No. 797).

References

1. Bomsel-Helmreich, O., Gougeon, A., Thebault, A., Saltarelli, D., Milgrom, E., Frydman, R. and Papiernik, E. (1979). Healthy and atretic human follicles in the preovulatory phase: differences in evolution of follicular morphology and steroid content of follicular fluid. *J. Clin. Endocrinol. Metab.*, **48**, 686–94
2. Koering, M. J. (1969). Cyclic changes in ovarian morphology during the menstrual cycle in *Macaca mulatta*. *Am. J. Anat.*, **126**, 73–101
3. Block, E. (1951). Quantitative morphological investigations of the follicular system in women. Variations in the different phases of the sexual cycle. *Acta Endocrinol.*, **8**, 33–59
4. Ross, G. T., Cargille, C. M., Lipsett, M. B., *et al.* (1970). Pituitary and gonadal hormones in women during spontaneous and induced ovulatory cycles. *Rec. Progr. Horm. Res.*, **26**, 1–62
5. Taymor, M. L., Berger, M. J., Thompson, I. E. and Karam, K. S. (1972). Hormonal factors in human ovulation. *Am. J. Obstet. Gynecol.*, **114**, 445–52
6. Dodson, K. S., Coutts, J. R. T. and MacNaughton, M. C. (1975). Plasma sex steroid and gonadotrophin patterns in human menstrual cycles. *Br. J. Obstet. Gynaecol.*, **82**, 602–14
7. Landgren, B. M. (1977). *Studies on the Pattern of Circulating Steroids in the Normal Menstrual Cycle*. PhD thesis, Stockholm
8. Corner, G. W. (1956). The histological dating of the human corpus luteum of menstruation. *Am. J. Anat.*, **98**, 377–401
9. Zeleznik, A. J., Midgley, A. R. and Reichert, L. E. (1974). Granulosa cell maturation in the rat: increased binding of human chorionic gonadotrophin following treatment with follicle-stimulating hormone *in vitro*. *Endocrinology*, **95**, 818–25
10. Richards, J. S. (1975). Estradiol receptor content in rat granulosa cells during follicular development: modification of estradiol and gonadotropins. *Endocrinology*, **97**, 1174–84

10a. Solari, A. (1977). Etude quantitative d'organes ou de tissus. III Méthode d'estimation du nombre de particules. *Ann. Biol. Anim. Biochim. Biophys.*, **17**, 309–24

11. Choudary, J. B., Gier, H. T. and Marion, G. B. (1968). Cyclic changes in bovine vesicular follicles. *J. Anim. Sci.*, **27**, 468–71

12. Brand, A. and de Jong, W. H. R. (1973). Qualitative and quantitative micromorphological investigations of the tertiary follicle population during the oestrous cycle in sheep. *J. Reprod. Fertil.*, **33**, 431–9

13. Greenwald, G. S. (1968). Influence of one or two ovaries on ovulation and ovarian weight in the hypophysectomized rat. *Endocrinology*, **82**, 591–6

14. Hirshfield, A. N. (1979). The role of FSH in the recruitment of large follicles. In Midgley, A. R. and Sadler, W. A. (eds.) *Ovarian Follicular Development and Function.* pp. 9–22. (New York: Raven Press)

15. Greenwald, G. S. (1961). Quantitative study of follicular development in the ovary of the intact or unilaterally ovariectomized hamster. *J. Reprod. Fertil.*, **2**, 351–61

16. Dufour, J., Cahill, L. P. and Mauleon, P. (1979). Short- and long-term effects of hypophysectomy and unilateral ovariectomy on ovarian follicular populations in sheep. *J. Reprod. Fertil.*, **57**, 301–9

17. Thibault, C. (1977). Are follicular maturation and oocyte maturation independent processes? *J. Reprod. Fertil.*, **51**, 1–15

18. Channing, C. P. and Batta, S. K. (1981). Follicular non steroidal regulators in women and sows. In Coutts, J. R. T. (ed.) *Functional Morphology of the Human Ovary.* pp. 73–84. (Lancaster: MTP Press)

19. Buffler, G. and Roser, S. (1974). New data concerning the role played by progesterone in the control of follicular growth in the rat. *Acta Endocrinol.*, **75**, 569–78

20. Goodman, A. L. and Hodgen, G. D. (1977). Systemic versus intraovarian replacement after luteectomy in rhesus monkeys: differential patterns of gonadotropins and follicle growth. *J. Clin. Endocrinol. Metab.*, **45**, 837–40

21. Gougeon, A. (1981). Rate of follicular growth in the human ovary. In *Follicular Maturation and Ovulation.* Proceedings of the IVth Reinier de Graaf Symposium. pp. 155–63. International Congress Series No. 560. (Amsterdam: Excerpta Medica)

22. Lunenfeld, B., Kraiem, Z. and Eshkol, A. (1976). Structure and function of the growing follicle. *Clin. Obstet. Gynecol.*, **3**, 27–42

23. Baird, D. T. and Fraser, I. S. (1975). Concentration of oestrone and oestradiol in follicular fluid and ovarian venous blood of women. *Clin. Endocrinol.*, **4**, 259–66

24. Peters, H. (1979). Discussion summary: session follicular development. In Midgley, A. R. and Sadler, W. A. (eds.) *Ovarian Follicular Development and Function.* pp. 39–40. (New York: Raven Press)

25. Richards, J. S. (1980). Maturation of ovarian follicles: actions and interactions of pituitary and ovarian hormones on follicular cell differentiation. *Physiol. Rev.*, **60**, 51–89

6
Hormonal control of Leydig cell function

J. M. Saez, M. Benahmed and J. Reventos

Testicular function is controlled by a complex, interacting system including the extrahypothalamic central nervous system, the hypothalamus, the pituitary gland and the gonads. Luteinizing hormone (LH) by interacting with specific receptors, is the main factor which regulates Leydig cell steroidogenesis while follicle stimulating hormone (FSH) controls Sertoli cell function. In turn, sex steroids produced by Leydig cells and the non-sex steroid factors of Sertoli cells modulate the peripheral concentrations of gonadotrophins. Recently, evidence has accumulated to indicate that many other hormones—including prolactin, LHRH, oestradiol, androgens, epidermal growth factor, neurohypophyseal hormones and catecholamines—can play a potential role in the regulation of Leydig cell function (reviewed in references 1 and 2). In addition, recent studies also suggest the existence of an important interaction between Leydig cells and the adjacent tubular cells resulting in the regulation of both Leydig and Sertoli cell functions.

This chapter is not intended to be an exhaustive literature review, but rather aims to highlight the potential physiological role of all these hormones on LH/hCG receptors of Leydig cells and on the steroidogenic capacity of these cells.

REGULATION OF TESTICULAR LH/hCG RECEPTORS

Factors which exert a positive effect on LH/hCG receptors

It seems that a normal pituitary function is necessary for the maintenance of the receptors. After hypophysectomy, there is rapid loss of LH receptors. The extent of this reduction varies widely according to different reports[3-6] and seems to be dependent on the age at which the hypophysectomy is performed[6,7]. There are several possible candidates as positive regulators of LH receptors.

FSH has been reported to have a positive effect on LH receptors of the testis, though the observed effects seem to be confined to the testis of immature hypophysectomized rats. Treatment of such rats with FSH results in a selective increase in testicular LH receptors which is accompanied by increased steroidogenic responsiveness to LH/hCG[8–10]. The effect of FSH was more marked on testicular steroidogenic responsiveness than on LH receptors, and could be inhibited by the simultaneous administration of oestrogens at doses that did not alter the FSH-induced increase in LH receptors[10–12]. However, there remains some unresolved questions concerning the role of FSH in the control of Leydig cell function and the mechanism by which its effects are exerted. Firstly, Purvis *et al.*[13] have suggested that the effects of FSH are due to small contaminations by LH, since neutralization of FSH with an LH antiserum abolishes the effects of FSH. These results, however, differ from those in other studies in which treatment with the expected quantity of LH contained in FSH had no effect on Leydig cell responsiveness[11]. Furthermore, the positive effects of ovine and bovine FSH were abolished following neuraminidase treatment of these preparations; such a treatment reduces the FSH activity but not that of the LH[14]. Secondly, the mechanism by which FSH exerts its effects on Leydig cell function is unknown, since FSH receptors have not been detected in these cells.

In a primary culture of crude testicular cells prepared from immature hypophysectomized rats, it has been reported that FSH alone had no effect on androgen production[15] but had a synergistic effect with hCG[16]. However, these synergistic effects were not observed by Verhoeven *et al.*[17] who used a primary culture containing mainly interstitial cells. Likewise, FSH treatment of cultured pig purified Leydig cells did not increase the number of LH/hCG receptors (Table 1), while the same treatment of crude Leydig cells containing Sertoli cells results in an increase in the number of LH/hCG receptors and accompanied by an increase in hCG-induced testosterone responses (Table 2). This suggests that the observed FSH effects on Leydig cell function are probably mediated via Sertoli cells.

The second pituitary hormone which has an important role in the control of LH receptors is prolactin. The positive effects of exogenous prolactin on testicular LH receptors has been shown in dwarf mice[24], seasonally regressed hamster[25]

Table 1 Effect of several hormones on [^{125}I]hCG binding and on the acute steroidogenic response to hCG of purified pig Leydig cells

Pretreatment	[^{125}I]hCG bound (% of control)	Testosterone (% of control)
Control	100 ± 6	100 ± 8
hCG (10^{-9} mol l^{-1})	5 ± 0.2	30 ± 2*
oFSH (20 ng ml^{-1})	104 ± 5	102 ± 9
oProlactin (500 ng ml^{-1})	99 ± 7	97 ± 5
EGF (10 ng ml^{-1})	85 ± 4*	92 ± 9
LHRH (10^{-7})	98 ± 7	104 ± 8
hLDL (40 μg ml^{-1})	82 ± 6*	616 ± 40*
hHDL (400 μg ml^{-1})	135 ± 7*	205 ± 18*
Oestradiol (10^{-7} mol l^{-1})	99 ± 8	102 ± 9

*$p < 0.05$ when compared with control.

Pig Leydig cells were prepared as described [18–22] and purified by a discontinuous Percoll gradient[23]. The cells were cultured in complete defined medium[18,19,21] without (control) or with the indicated factors for 3 days. The medium was changed daily. On the third day some dishes were used to measure the specific binding of [^{125}I]hCG, the others were treated with hCG 3×10^{-9} mol l^{-1} for 4 h to measure testosterone production. The results are expressed as percentage of control ([^{125}I]hCG binding, 5×10^4 cpm/10^6 cells; testosterone production, 18 ± 2 ng/10^6 cells/4 h).

Table 2 Effects of FSH on crude Leydig cells and purified Leydig cells specific activities

Variable	Crude Leydig cells FSH (ng ml^{-1})			Purified Leydig cells FSH (ng ml^{-1})		
	0	50	100	0	50	100
[^{125}I]hCG binding (% of control)	100 ± 7	129 ± 5	141 ± 6	100 ± 6	97 ± 6	104 ± 8
Testosterone (ng/day/dish):						
Basal	1.7 ± 0.4	1.8 ± 0.6	2.3 ± 0.8	2.6 ± 0.4	2.1 ± 0.2	2.5 ± 0.5
hCG	35 ± 3	46 ± 5	62 ± 6	46 ± 4	44 ± 3	49 ± 5

Crude Leydig cells and purified Leydig cells prepared as indicated in Table 1 were cultured for 3 days in the absence of LDL with or without the indicated concentration of oFSH. On the last day of culture, some dishes received hCG (10^{-9} mol l^{-1}).

75

hypophysectomized rats[4,10,24] and intact adult male rats[26]. Also, in intact animals, induction of hyperprolactinaemia leads to increased testicular LH/hCG receptors[27,28]. Conversely, reduction of plasma prolactin levels by treatment with 2-bromo-α-ergocryptine causes a decrease in testicular LH/hCG receptors[26,29,30]. Although Leydig cells contain specific prolactin receptors[31], the mechanisms by which this hormone exerts its positive effects on LH receptors are not clear. In intact rats, it has been suggested that the increase in LH receptors may be a consequence of a lower rate of LH receptor loss, which in turn is due to the chronic reduction in circulating levels of LH very often present in hyperprolactinaemia[28]. However, in hypophysectomized animals, prolactin must exert its effects on Leydig cells either by causing an increase of LH receptor synthesis or a decrease of degradation, but it is still unclear whether the effects are due to a direct interaction between the hormone and Leydig cells or whether they are mediated indirectly through other testicular cell types. In favour of the latter hypothesis is the lack of effect of prolactin on LH receptors of cultured purified Leydig cells (Table 1).

Several workers have proposed that GH could also exert a positive effect on Leydig cell LH receptors. Hence, GH administration to hypophysectomized rats prevents to some extent the spontaneous loss of LH receptors[4,5]. The effects of GH and prolactin are additive, which suggests that they are probably acting at different sites in the rat testis[4]. In addition, prolactin treatment of hypophysectomized rats allowed low doses of LH to have a positive effect on its receptors and partially prevented the LH-induced loss of LH/hCG receptors, while GH treatment had no such effects[4]. On the other hand GH had a positive effect on testicular steroidogenic responsiveness to LH, while prolactin did not.

At low concentrations, the positive effects of LH on its own receptors have been demonstrated by the fact that, after hypophysectomy, the LH receptor loss was completely prevented if low doses of LH were added to GH and prolactin treatment[4,5]. However, LH alone at higher doses induced a further decrease in LH receptors. Likewise, in cultured pig Leydig cells[19] and in mouse Leydig cell tumour[32,33], LH or hCG, even at low concentrations, always induces 'down-regulation' of its own receptors (see below).

Experimental diabetes in male rats is often accompanied by a marked decrease in testicular steroidogenesis, which is due to the impairment of both pituitary and gonadal functions[34]. In the same experimental model, testicular LH/hCG receptors are decreased, and insulin administration to diabetic animals restores the binding capacity to normal values, indicating that insulin might have a positive effect on LH receptors[35]. In vitro, insulin has a synergetic effect with hCG on androgen production by cultured rat testicular cells[36]. However, this effect seems to be exerted at a point distal to receptor, since insulin also enhances the steroidogenic response to dibutyryl cAMP and choleragen[36]. In cultured rat testicular cells this effect of insulin on steroidogenesis seems to be specific and independent of an overall enhancement of testicular metabolic function[36], while in cultured pig Leydig cells insulin is absolutely required for cell survival[19,20].

Another factor which, in vitro, produces an increase in the number of LH/hCG receptors on cultured pig Leydig cells, is human HDL (Table 1). In contrast, human LDL produces a small but significant decrease of LH receptors (Table 1). However, both LDL and HDL enhance the steroidogenic response to hCG, although the effect of LDL is far higher than that of HDL (Table 1).

Factors which exert a negative effect on LH/hCG receptors

hCG-induced receptor loss

Like other membrane-bound hormones, LH and hCG have the ability to regulate negatively the number of their own receptors on Leydig cells. The regulation of gonadotrophin receptors by LH or hCG has been documented *in vivo*[1,3,37] and *in vitro* using Leydig cells from normal[19,20,38] and tumoural tissues[32,33,39]. Within the first hours of gonadotrophin administration to male rat, there is a small transient increase of LH binding sites[40] and this increase seems to be dependent on intact microfilament and steroidogenesis. However, this increase has not been observed in *in vitro* studies using mouse[32,33] or pig[19] Leydig cells. Thereafter, *in vivo*, there is a dose- and time-dependent decrease of the apparent number of binding sites (Figure 1(*a*)). This intial loss of LH binding capacity is due to

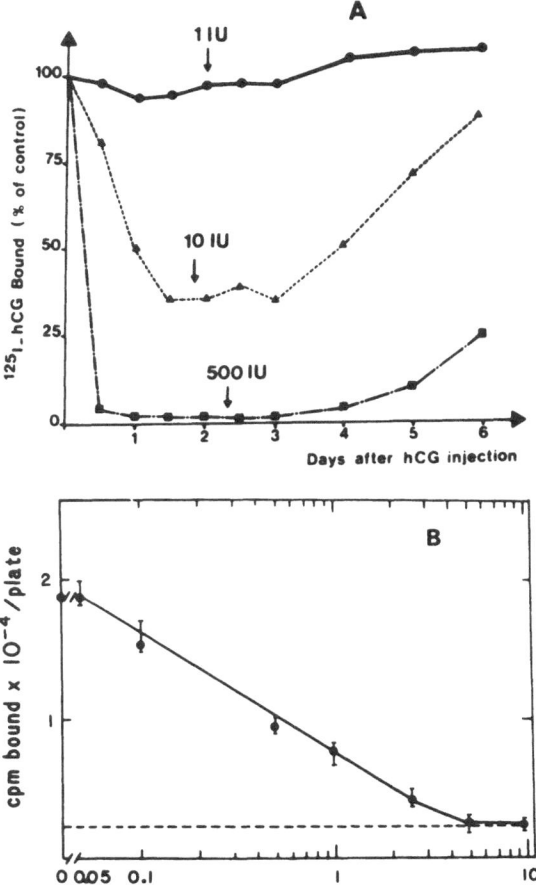

Figure 1 (*a*) Effect of a single injection of different doses of hCG to adult male rats on the number of hCG binding sites of interstitial cell particles prepared from isolated rat Leydig cells. (*b*) Effect of different doses of hCG on the apparent number of hCG receptors of cultured pig Leydig cells. The number of binding sites (cpm/10⁶ cells) were measured 24 h after the addition of hCG (Reproduced from reference 19, by permission of publishers.)

occupancy of receptors by the dose of the injected hormone[41]. *In vitro*, hCG also induces an apparent receptor loss, dose- and time-dependent, in cultured pig Leydig cells[19] (Figure 1(*b*)). However, as observed *in vivo*, more than 50% of the apparent receptor loss during the first day is due to occupancy[19,21]. On the contrary, in a mouse tumour Leydig cell line[32,39] the hCG-induced decrease in binding capacity seems to be related almost exclusively to receptor loss. The receptor loss requires protein synthesis since cycloheximide blocks the process both *in vivo*[42] and *in vitro*[33]. Autoradiographic and immunofluorescent studies suggest that some plasma membrane-associated hCG receptor complexes are translocated within the cells, where the hormone is degraded[32,39,43–45]. The rate of this process is very fast in mouse tumour Leydig cells[32,39,43], since most of the bound hormone is internalized and degraded within 6 h. On the contrary, in normal rat[46] and in cultured pig Leydig cells[47], some of the hormone–receptor complexes are still visible at the membrane level several days following hormonal removal, suggesting that the internalization process in these cases is very slow. The rate of gonadotrophin receptor replenishment in normal Leydig cells after extensive 'down regulation' is relatively slow both *in vivo* (Figure 1) and *in vitro*[48] and takes several days before the normal complement of sites is recovered.

Effect of LHRH and its analogues

The hypothalamic peptide LHRH is the main factor regulating the secretion of gonadotrophins by the anterior pituitary and therefore the gonadal function. However, chronic administration of LHRH or its agonists to male rats induces a decrease of the testicular LH receptor content[26,49,50]. Since the inhibitory effects of LHRH agonists on gonadal function are parallel to their LH-releasing potency[50], the effects observed have been initially attributed to the release of endogenous LH, with secondary testicular desensitization[26,49,50]. However, in the last few years it has been demonstrated that LHRH agonists have extra-pituitary effects, in particular a direct action at the gonadal level (review in reference 51). Hence, a direct effect of LHRH agonists on testicular function has been suggested by the ability of these compounds to reduce the number of testicular LH/hCG receptors in immature and hypophysectomized rats[52] and to block the FSH-induced increase in testicular weight, LH/hCG receptors and steroidogenic responsiveness to gonadotrophins, in hypophysectomized rats[10,53]. Since rat Leydig cells contain specific LHRH binding sites[51], the above results suggest that the inhibitory effect of this peptide on testicular function is mediated by its interaction with Leydig cells. In favour of this hypothesis is the inhibitory effect of LHRH analogues on hCG-induced androgen production by cultured rat testicular cells[17,54]. These inhibitory effects of LHRH agonists are observed both *in vivo* and *in vitro* after a lag period of about 1–2 days. In addition, it has recently been shown that LHRH agonists, after an initial lag period of about 2 h, produce a marked stimulation of testosterone production over a 32 h period[55–58]. These studies indicate that the mechanism of both stimulatory and inhibitory effects of LHRH on rat Leydig cell functions are distinct from the stimulatory and de-sensitizing effects of hCG which require a shorter time course of action. However, the main question concerning the effect of LHRH analogues on testicular function is to know whether the results observed in rats can be extrapolated to other species. From the available data, this does not seem to be the case. Firstly, neither mouse Leydig[57] nor human interstitial cells[59] contain specific binding sites for

LHRH; secondly, in a mouse Leydig cell line[60], in normal cultured mouse Leydig cells[57] and in cultured pig Leydig cells (Table 1)[21], LHRH agonists had neither the initial stimulatory effect on testicular androgen production, nor the long-term inhibitory effect on hCG-induced androgen production.

EGF

Another factor which produces an apparent loss of LH/hCG receptors *in vitro* is EGF. In a clonal strain of mouse Leydig tumour cells, low concentrations of EGF induced an 80–90% reduction in the number of hCG receptors and a decrease in the steroidogenic response to hCG but not to 8-bromo-cAMP[61]. In cultured pig Leydig cells, however, the effect of EGF on hCG receptors is far less pronounced and is not accompanied by a corresponding reduction of the steroidogenic capacity (Table 1).

REGULATION OF TESTICULAR STEROIDOGENESIS

Factors which increase the steroidogenic capacity of Leydig cells

The steroidogenic function of the Leydig cells is primarily maintained by LH probably in synergism with other pituitary hormones such as FSH, prolactin and growth hormone. Under physiological conditions, the role of LH is double: immediate regulation of testosterone production and trophic effects responsible for maintenance of several enzymatic activities in the steroidogenic pathway. The first effect is due to an increased conversion of cholesterol to pregnenolone, which is the rate-limiting step in steroidogenesis and is mediated by an activation of cytochrome P-450[62]. This activation is the final step of the pathway which starts with the binding of the hormone to its receptor and involves increased formation of cAMP, activation of the protein kinases, protein synthesis, activation of phospholipids metabolism and finally translocation of cholesterol to the inner membrane of mitochondria[62–66].

The trophic effect of LH on Leydig cells has been inferred by the rapid decline, following hypophysectomy, in almost all the key enzymes of the steroidogenic pathway, particularly in cholesterol side-chain cleavage activity[67] and the recovery of the steroidogenic capacity following treatment with small doses of LH for a few days[4]. It is interesting to note that treatment of hypophysectomized rats with FSH completely restores the capacity of Leydig cells to produce pregnenolone following LH stimulation[67] while the ability to produce testosterone is only partially restored[4, 67].

Leydig cells, like other steroidogenic cells, require cholesterol for steroid hormone production. Cholesterol can be synthetized *de novo* from acetate[68] or can enter the cells as a component of the plasma lipoproteins[69]. Recent work from several laboratories has demonstrated that the bulk of the cholesterol utilized for the synthesis of steroids in adrenals[70, 71], ovaries[72] and placenta[73] originates from plasma lipoproteins, mainly low density lipoprotein (LDL), except in the rat which preferentially utilizes high density lipoprotein (HDL). The reported results concerning the origin of cholesterol utilized by Leydig cells are contradictory. The data of Morris *et al.*[74] indicate that most cholesterol used for androgen synthesis in rat testis is derived from *de novo* synthesis while the data of Anderson *et al.*[75] using an *in vivo* hypocholesterolaemic rat model suggest that cholesterol from HDL is the major substrate for testosterone production. *In vitro* studies have confirmed and extended these data. Rat interstitial tissue contains specific binding sites for human HDL[76], and HDL increases the rate of testosterone production of cultured rat testicular cells[77]. Likewise, cultured pig Leydig cells contain specific binding sites for human LDL[78], and addition of this lipoprotein to the incubation medium increases the steroidogenic capacity of Leydig cells (Figure 2). The effects of LDL are more effective than those of HDL despite the fact that HDL increases the number of hCG receptors. The data shown in Figure 2 clearly indicates that the effects of lipoprotein and hCG are synergistic, since steroid production by concomitant treatment with hCG and lipoproteins was more important than the sum of each added individually.

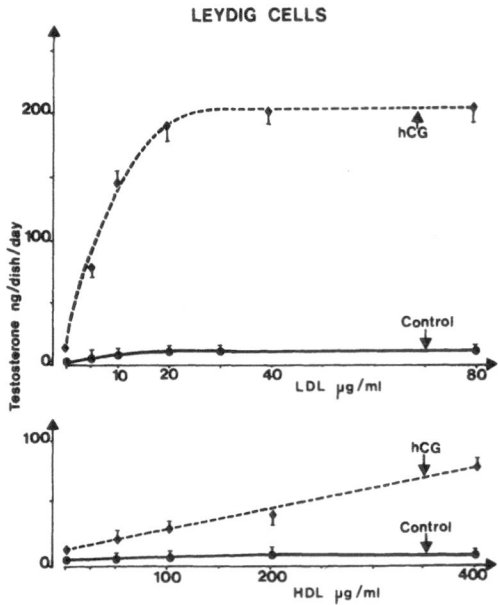

Figure 2 Effects of human lipoproteins LDL and HDL and hCG on testosterone production by purified pig Leydig cells. Cells were cultured for 3 days without (control) or with hCG (10^{-9} mol l^{-1}) in the presence of indicated concentration of lipoproteins. The medium was changed daily and testosterone was measured in the medium of the 3rd day

As indicated above, *in vivo* studies indicate that several hormones, FSH, prolactin and GH increase the steroidogenic responsiveness of Leydig cells to hCG. This effect can be in part related to an increase in the number of hCG binding sites. In addition to this effect on hCG receptors, these hormones seem to increase the activity of some enzymes in steroidogenesis[67, 79]. On the other hand, the mechanism by which these hormones enhance Leydig cell function is not well understood. Concerning FSH, no receptors for this hormone have been detected on Leydig cells, and it has no effect on the steroidogenesis of cultured purified pig Leydig cells (Tables 1 and 2) but clearly increases the steroidogenic response to hCG of cultured crude pig Leydig cells containing about 40% Sertoli cells (Table 2). A synergistic effect of FSH and hCG has been also observed in a primary culture of total rat interstitial cells[16, 80]. These results indicate that the effects of FSH on Leydig function are probably mediated by Sertoli cells. This hypothesis has been confirmed in this laboratory using a co-culture of purified pig Leydig and Sertoli cells (Figure 3)[21].

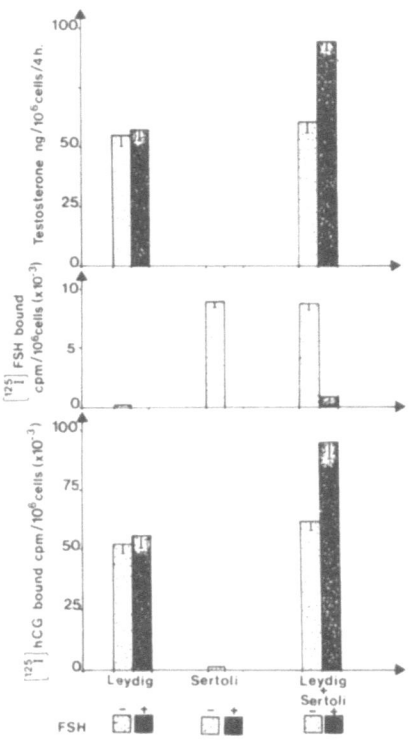

Figure 3 Effects of co-culture of purified pig Leydig cells with purified pig Sertoli cells on the specific function of Leydig cells. Leydig and Sertoli cells were cultured separately or together (Leydig/Sertoli rates: 1:4) for 3 days in the presence or absence of oFSH (50 ng ml^{-1}). On the last day the specific binding of [^{125}I]hCG (bottom panel), of [^{125}I]FSH (middle panel) and the acute steroidogenic response to hCG (10^{-9} mol l^{-1}) were measured

Specific prolactin receptors are present in rat Leydig cells[31] and as indicated above, prolactin increases both the number of hCG receptors and the steroidogenic response to hCG of rodent testis *in vivo*. However, *in vitro*, prolactin has no effect on either hCG binding sites or steroidogenic capacity of cultured purified pig Leydig cells (Table 1). This discrepancy between the *in vivo* and *in vitro* results could be due to differences in the species studied or to the fact that the stimulatory effects of prolactin are exerted through adjacent testicular cells that in turn influence the Leydig cells.

Several years ago it was reported that testosterone synthesis in perfused dog testis could be stimulated by β-adrenergic agonist[81]. More recently it has been shown that these compounds are able to stimulate cAMP and testosterone production by cultured purified mouse Leydig cells[82], but have no effect on fresh isolated cells. The possible physiological role of catecholamines on the regulation of testosterone production *in vivo* is unknown.

Factors which decrease the steroidogenic capacity of Leydig cells

hCG-induced desensitization

As discussed above, small doses of LH or hCG have a positive effect on the steroidogenic capacity of Leydig cells *in vivo*. However, high levels of LH or hCG have deleterious effects on the characteristics of the Leydig cell response to further gonadotrophin stimulation. Several laboratories have shown (reviewed in references 1 and 2) that in rats, following the initial stimulation of cAMP and steroid production induced by high doses of LH or hCG, testicular cells soon become resistant to further hormonal stimulation (Figure 4). This refractoriness

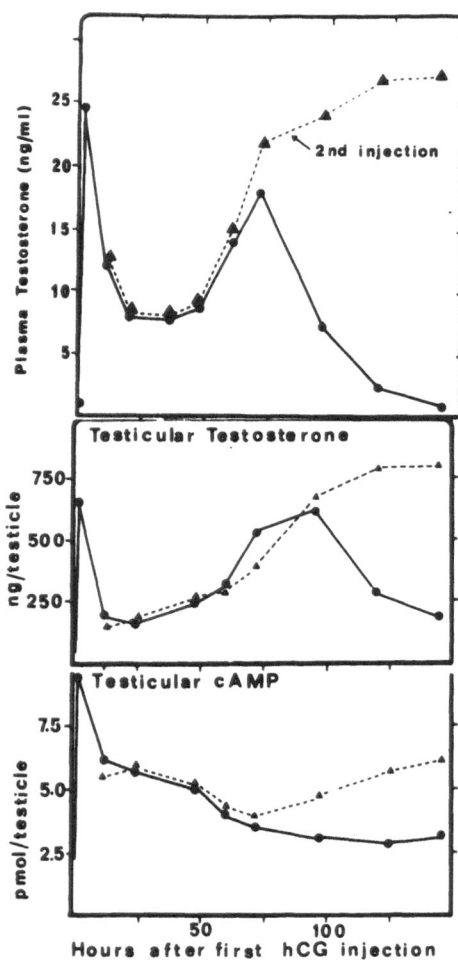

Figure 4 Effect of a single injection of 500 IU of hCG on plasma testosterone (top panel), testicular testosterone (middle panel) and testicular cAMP (bottom panel) content. At the time indicated, half of the animals were injected with saline (●) while the other half received a second injection of 500 IU of hCG (▲ ... ▲). Animals were killed 2 h later

or desensitization was initially related to the loss of receptors[41]. However, further *in vivo* studies clearly demonstrate that the time course of LH/hCG receptor loss and of desensitization, as well as the doses of hormone required to induce both phenomena, were different[4,42,83,84]. Within the first hours of hCG administration, the steroidogenic refractoriness seems to be related mainly to a lack of hormone activation of adenylate cyclase[42,85,86]. This desensitization seems to be related to some alteration of the N subunit of the enzyme, since hormonal responsiveness is restored by addition of human erythrocyte extracts (containing the N subunit) to interstitial cell membranes prepared from hCG-desensitized testes[86]. However, changes in the LH receptor and the adenylate cyclase activity cannot entirely explain the hCG-induced steroidogenic refractoriness, since desensitized cells also become resistant to the steroidogenic effects of cholera toxin and dibutyryl cAMP, as shown in Figure 5[84,87,88]. This steroidogenic refractoriness to exogenous and endogenous cAMP is not due to a modification of either phosphodiesterases[84]

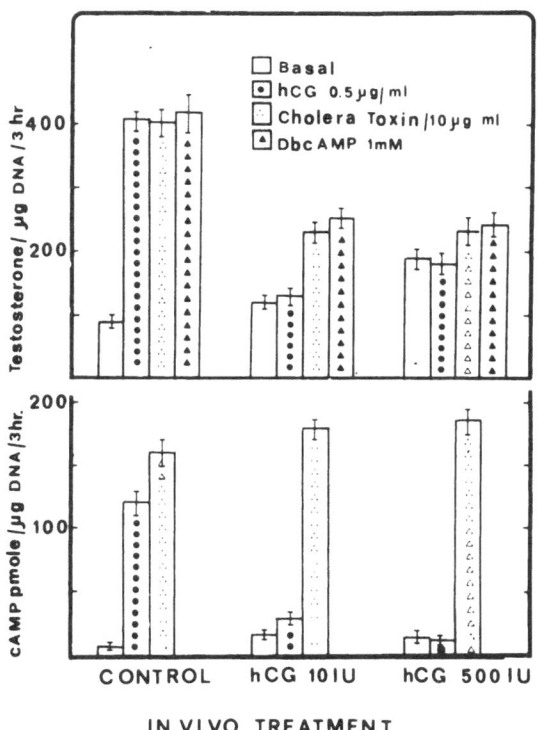

Figure 5 *In vitro* cAMP and testosterone response to several stimuli of isolated Leydig cells from rats treated with different doses of hCG 36 h before

or cAMP-dependent protein kinase[88] activities. The main alterations of the steroidogenic pathway during cell desensitization are a decrease of 17α-hydroxylase and 17-20-lyase activities (Figure 6)[84,87–90]. After high doses of hCG, in addition to these alterations, there is also a decreased pregnenolone formation[88,91,92]. The desensitizing effects of high doses of hCG have also been observed in several animal species[93,94] as well as in man[95,96]. The profile of plasma testosterone in man after hCG administration (Figure 7) is similar to that observed in rats (Figure 4).

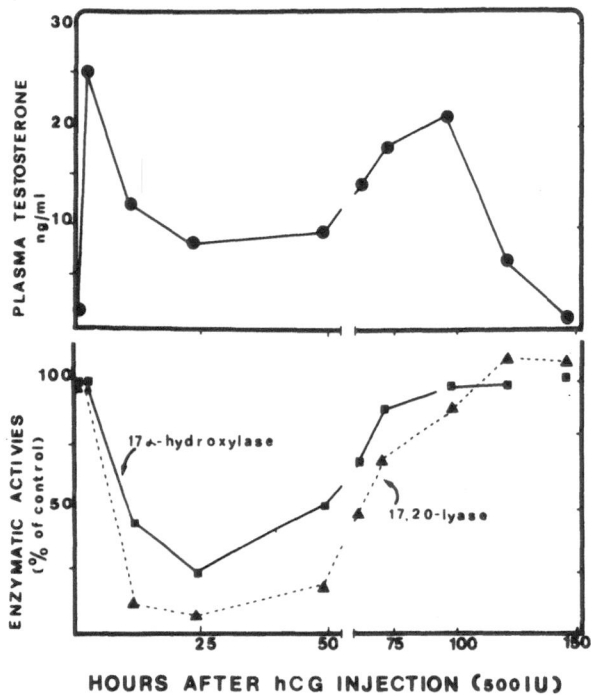

HOURS AFTER hCG INJECTION (500IU)

Figure 6 Effects of a single injection of 500 IU hCG to adult rats on plasma testosterone levels (top panel) and on microsomal 17α-hydroxylase and 17-20 lyase testicular activities (lower panel)

All the above data indicate that the hCG-induced Leydig cell steroidogenic desensitization is a complex process due to several phenomena which include: loss of LH receptors, alteration of the coupling between the receptor and the adenylate cyclase, decreased formation of pregnenolone and decreased 17α-hydroxylase and 17-20 lyase activities. It has been reported that the decreased formation of pregnenolone in rat testis is observed only after the administration of high doses of hCG[87,97]. However, in a mouse Leydig cell line which mainly secretes progesterone[32,39,61], hCG at low concentrations and dibutyryl cAMP induce desensitization of the steroidogenic response to hCG, dibutyryl cAMP and cholera toxin[32]. Likewise, hCG and dibutyryl cAMP treatment of purified pig Leydig cells in culture produce heterologous steroidogenic refractoriness to the stimulatory effects of both substances (Figure 8)[21]. Since dibutyryl cAMP did not produce loss of LH receptors in both the mouse and the pig models, the results indicate that the lesions responsible for the steroidogenic refractoriness must be located beyond cAMP formation and that it is not related to LH receptor loss.

The decreased steroidogenic capacity of desensitized rat Leydig cells could be due to a depletion of the cholesterol available for steroidogenesis. Indeed, it has been reported that the *in vitro* steroidogenic responsiveness of rat desensitized

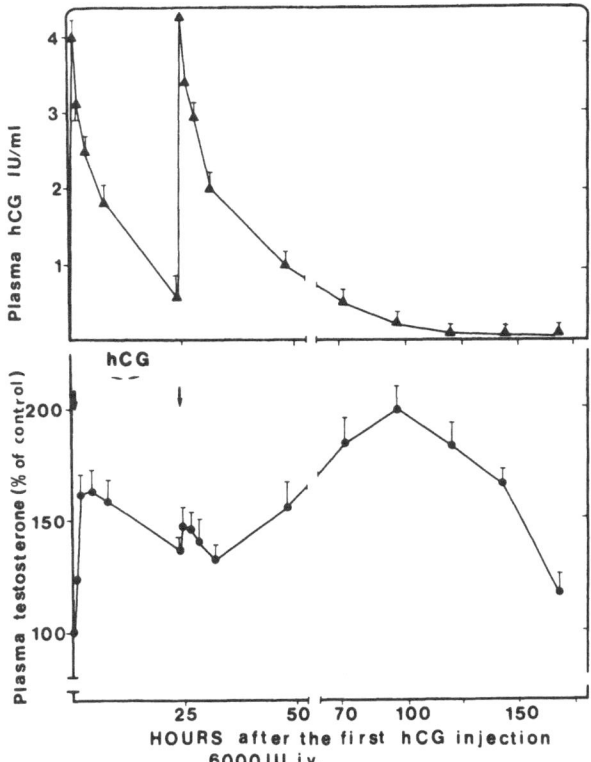

Figure 7 Effects in man of two successive i.v. injections of 6000 IU hCG administered with a 24 h interval on the plasma levels of several steroids (Reproduced from reference 96, with permission of publishers.)

Leydig cells was completely restored by addition of HDL or LDL[98]. However, this cholesterol depletion seems not to be the sole explanation of steroidogenic refractoriness, since even high concentrations of LDL only partially prevent hCG- and dibutyryl cAMP-induced steroidogenic desensitization in cultured pig Leydig cells (Figure 8)[21].

Data from several laboratories have suggested that the decreased activity of 17α-hydroxylase and 17-20 lyase observed in rat Leydig cells following *in vivo* administration of hCG could be mediated by oestradiol. Firstly, administration of oestrogens to rats produced a decreased steroidogenic capacity of Leydig cells, which has been related to a decreased activity of both enzymes[92, 97, 99]. Secondly, testicular oestradiol levels increase after i.v. injection of hCG[100–102]. Thirdly, following the injection of hCG, there is a depletion of the oestradiol cytosol receptor, and its translocation to the nucleus, both phenomena occur in parallel with the increase in the oestrogen concentration of the testis[101–103]. Finally, administration of an anti-oestrogen (tamoxifen) before hCG prevents the hCG-induced steroidogenic desensitization[99, 101].

Recent data, however, have cast some doubt on the role of oestradiol in these enzymatic alterations which produce inhibition of Leydig cell steroidogenesis:

85

(1) depletion of the cytosol receptor concentration does not always result in an inhibition of testicular steroidogenesis[92, 104]; (2) the time course of oestradiol receptor depletion and 17-20 lyase inhibition following hCG or oestradiol administration does not fit very well with that hypothesis[90]; (3) in contrast to the results cited above which showed that tamoxifen can block hCG-induced steroidogenic desensitization[100, 102], other workers were unable to confirm these results[103]; (4) if it is true that oestradiol at very high concentrations (10^{-6}–10^{-5} mol l^{-1}) inhibits rat Leydig cell steroidogenesis[105] these concentrations are probably never reached *in vivo*[90].

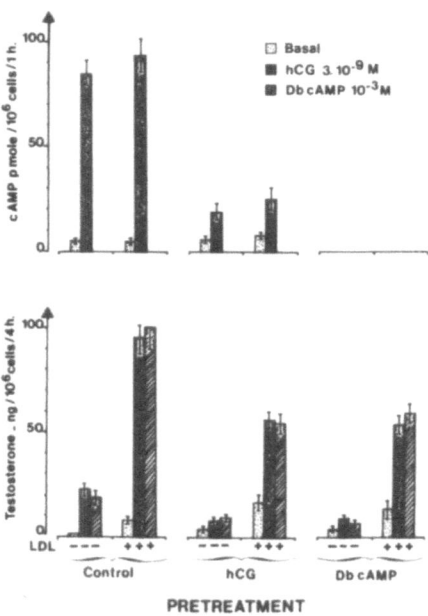

Figure 8 Effects of human LDL, hCG and dibutyryl cAMP treatment on pig Leydig cells activities. Purified pig Leydig cells were cultured for 3 days in the absence or presence of hCG (10^{-9} mol l^{-1}) dibutyryl cAMP (10^{-3} mol l^{-1}) and hLDL (20 µg ml^{-1}). The medium was changed daily. On the 3rd day the medium was removed and fresh medium was added with or without hCG (3×10^{-9} mol l^{-1}) or dibutyryl cAMP (10^{-3} mol l^{-1}). cAMP and testosterone were measured in the medium 1 and 4 h later, respectively

More recently, in a primary culture of crude rat interstitial cells, it has been shown[38] that hCG (3×10^{-10}–3×10^{-8} mol l^{-1}) induced the same steroidogenic lesions as that observed following hCG administration *in vivo*. The addition of tamoxifen 20 min prior to hCG treatment completely prevents the lesion of 17α-hydroxylase/17-20 lyase. In the same study, it was reported that treatment of cultured cells with oestradiol (4×10^{-9}–4×10^{-7} mol l^{-1}) induced a decrease in the activity of both 17α-hydroxylase and 17-20 lyase. Such lesions were prevented by tamoxifen treatment of cultured cells prior to the addition of oestrogens[38]. In contrast to these results, are the lack of effect of oestradiol even at high concentrations (10^{-6} mol l^{-1}) on the steroidogenesis of cultured mouse[106] and pig[22] (Figure 9) Leydig cells. It must be noted that hCG induces steroidogenic desensitization of cultured pig Leydig cells (Figure 9) and that these cells contain specific cytosol oestradiol receptors which are translocated to the nucleus by oestradiol[22].

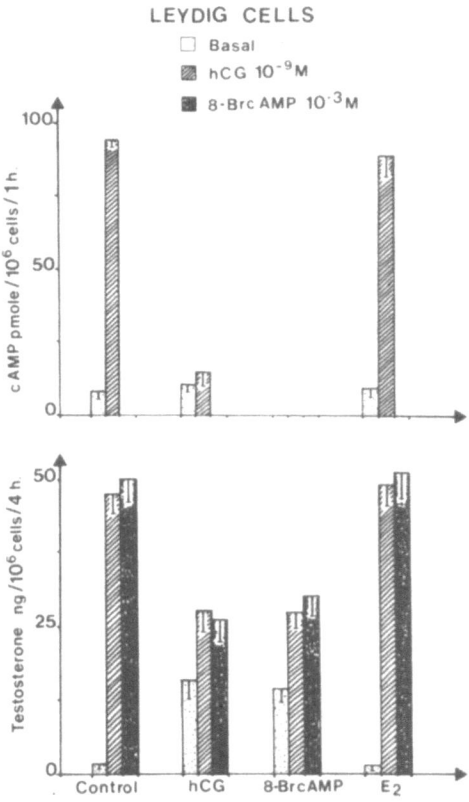

Figure 9 Effects of hCG ($10^{-9}\,\mathrm{mol\,l^{-1}}$), dibutyryl cAMP ($10^{-3}\,\mathrm{mol\,l^{-1}}$) and oestradiol ($E_2$) ($10^{-6}\,\mathrm{mol\,l^{-1}}$) on purified pig Leydig cell steroidogenesis responsiveness. The conditions were similar to those described in Figure 8. LDL was present ($20\,\mu\mathrm{g\,ml^{-1}}$)

The discrepancy between the inhibitory effect of oestradiol on cultured rat interstitial cells and the lack of effects on cultured mouse and pig Leydig cells are related either to differences between species or between models used. The first hypothesis is not unlikely, since the response of rat Leydig cells to other hormones is different from that of mouse and pig Leydig cells: i.e. rat Leydig cells contain specific LHRH receptor[51] and this peptide induces an initial short-term stimulation of steroidogenesis[55–59] and thereafter steroidogenic desensitization[16,54], while mouse Leydig cells do not contain LHRH receptors and the peptide has neither stimulatory nor inhibitory effect on the steroidogenesis of these cells as for pig Leydig cells, in the latter case[21,57]. The differences in the model could also contribute to explaining this discrepancy. In the rat model, the culture contained crude interstitial cells (10–20% Leydig cells) while in the pig model more than 95% of cells in culture were Leydig cells[22]. Therefore one can postulate that the effects of oestradiol might be exerted through adjacent testicular cells, which could be present in crude rat cultured interstitial cells but not in purified Leydig cells.

Inhibitory effect of other hormones on Leydig cell steroidogenesis

Work from many laboratories has clearly shown that in several physiological or pathological conditions, testicular androgen production can be modified without significant changes in the plasma levels of gonadotrophins[107]. Investigations carried out during the last decade have tried to highlight the factor(s) able to modify Leydig cell steroidogenic capacity. It must be pointed out that most of these studies have been performed using the rat model.

Chronic psychological or somatic stress induces a decrease in plasma testosterone levels[108,109]. The decrease in plasma testosterone levels was initially related to a decreased LH secretion, but it has recently been shown that decreased testosterone levels may occur in stressed animals with normal levels of LH[109] and decreased response to low dose of hCG[110]. Moreover, the steroidogenic response of interstitial cells isolated from stressed animals to hCG and dibutyryl cAMP was decreased, indicating that the lesion must be located beyond cAMP formation. However, the factors responsible for such alteration remain unknown.

High levels of glucocorticoids produce a decrease in plasma testosterone levels in man[111] and in rats[112] and lower responses to hCG stimulation. This partial refractoriness seems to be related to a decrease in the number of testicular LH receptors[112,113]. Recent *in vitro* studies have confirmed that glucocorticoids inhibit the hCG-stimulated androgen production in rat interstitial cells[113] and in pig purified Leydig cells[114]. However, as in the case of stress, the lesions responsible for this steroidogenic refractoriness have as yet not been demonstrated.

In vivo studies have suggested that rat testicular testosterone production may be controlled via a short-loop testosterone negative feedback mechanism[115,116]. In favour of this hypothesis is the observation that infusion of testosterone into the testicular artery of the rat inhibits LH-stimulated testosterone secretion[116]. Both the inhibition and the recovery of testosterone secretion are very rapid[116] suggesting that testosterone or its metabolites exert their effects by competitive inhibition. This short-loop negative feedback could also be the explanation of the time-course response of cultured pig Leydig cells to hCG: the response is linear for about 12 h but thereafter slows down. However, if after 16 h of hCG stimulation, the medium is removed and replaced by fresh medium, the cells respond again as well as during the period of the first incubation[21,117]. This indicates that hCG induces the excretion and accumulation of some products by Leydig cells, which in turn inhibit testosterone secretion. In addition to this rapid-short negative feedback, it has been reported that an androgen-agonist (R 1881) can inhibit the steroidogenic effect of hCG, dibutyryl cAMP and cholera toxin on rat interstitial cells in culture[118]. On the contrary, an androgen antagonist (cyproterone acetate) increased the steroidogenic effects of the three substances. Although the time courses of effects of androgen agonists and antagonists have not been determined, it is likely that these effects are mediated by specific receptors.

As indicated above, EGF at low concentrations produces a loss of LH/hCG receptors in a clonal strain of murine Leydig tumour cells[61]. The loss of hCG receptors is accompanied by a corresponding reduction in the ability of hCG to stimulate progesterone production by these cells which lack the androgen biosynthetic capacity. However, the steroidogenic responses to cholera toxin and 8-bromo-cAMP are not affected. The effect of EGF on hCG receptors of cultured pig Leydig cells is far less pronounced (Table 1) and this effect is not accompanied by a reduction of the steroidogenic response to hCG. In contrast, EGF inhibits significantly hCG-, dibutyryl cAMP-, and cholera toxin-stimulated testosterone production by a primary culture of crude rat testicular cells[119, 120]. This inhibition seems to be related to a decreased activity of 17α-hydroxylase and 17-20 lyase[120].

The antigonadal effects of neurohypophyseal hormone have been described in rodents[121] and in dogs[122]. These effects could be indirect and mediated by the suppression of gonadotrophin release by the neurohypophysial hormone[123]. More recently, however, it has been shown that vasopressin and related neuro-hypophysial hormones inhibit hCG-, dibutyryl cAMP- and cholera toxin-stimulated testosterone production in a primary culture of crude rat testicular cells[124, 125]. As in the case of EGF, the inhibition seems to be mainly due to selective suppression of the enzymes 17α-hydroxylase and 17-20 lyase[125].

CONCLUDING REMARKS

In vivo, Leydig cell function is undoubtedly controlled mainly by LH. However, it is clear that many other hormones can modulate the responsiveness of these cells to gonadotrophin stimulation. Evidence has accumulated to indicate that Leydig-Sertoli cell interactions play a key role not only in the development and function of the seminiferous tubules[126] but also in the function of Leydig cells[126–128]. The data reported here clearly indicate that the positive effect of FSH on Leydig cell steroidogenic capacity is mediated by Sertoli cells, but that the factor(s) responsible for such effects are still unknown. Likewise, it is not unlikely that the effects of other hormones on Leydig cell steroidogenesis might be exerted through adjacent testicular cells that in turn influence Leydig cell function. This hypothesis could explain the surprising observation that the same steroidogenic impairments of rat Leydig cells (decreased 17α-hydroxylase and 17-20 lyase activities) have been found *in vivo* after administration of hCG[86, 89], LHRH[1] and arginine–vasotocin[129] and *in vitro* after treatment of cultured rat interstitial cells with hCG[38], EGF[120], oestradiol[38] and arginine–vasotocin[125]. Thus a tentative explanation is that the inhibitory effect of all these hormones on Leydig cell steroidogenesis could be mediated by the same factor(s) secreted by other testicular cell types. The goal for future research should be to try working with purified preparations containing each testicular cell type, or in combinations of these in order to determine the effects of each hormone and the interaction between hormones in a particular cell type, and between cells.

The second pitfall in our understanding of Leydig cell regulation comes from the fact that the majority of studies concerning this problem have been performed using rat testis. Several observations indicate, however, that the steroidogenic pathway, the steroidogenic capacity and the volume and surface of cytoplasmic organelles of rat Leydig cells are different from those of other mammalian testes[130–132]. More intriguing are the differences between the inhibitory effect of some factors (oestradiol, EGF, LHRH) on rat Leydig cell steroidogenesis and the absence of effect of these factors in other species (pig, mouse). These observations provoke the question whether the rat testicular model is representative of most mammalian testes.

Acknowledgements

The results reported were supported by a grant from le Ministère de la Recherche et de l'Industrie (no. 82-L-0853) and a grant from la Fondation pour la Recherche Médicale Française. The authors thank Miss Joëlle Bois for her faithful secretarial assistance.

References

1. Catt, K. J., Harwood, J. P., Clayton, R. N., et al. (1980). Rec. Prog. Horm. Res., 36, 557–622
2. Saez, J. M. and Benahmed, M. (1984). In Posner, B. I. (ed.) Polypeptide Hormone Receptors. (In press) (New York: Marcel Dekker)
3. Haour, F., Sanchez, P., Cathiard, A. M. and Saez, J. M. (1978). Biochem. Biophys. Res. Commun., 81, 547–51
4. Payne, A. H. and Zipf, W. B. (1978). Intern. J. Androl. Suppl., 2, 329–44
5. Zipf, W. B., Payne, A. H. and Kelch, R. P. (1978). Endocrinology, 103, 595–600
6. Purvis, K., Clausen, O. P. F. and Hansson, V. (1980). J. Reprod. Fertil., 60, 77–86
7. Purvis, K., Clausen, O. P. F., Torjesen, P. A. and Hansson, U. (1979). Int. J. Androl., 2, 74–85
8. Odell, W. D. and Swerdloff, R. S. (1976). Rec. Prog. Horm. Res., 32, 245–88
9. Chen, Y. D. I., Shaw, M. J. and Payne, A. H. (1977). Mol. Cell. Endocrinol., 8, 291–9
10. Bambino, T. H., Schreiber, J. R. and Hsueh, A. J. W. (1980). Endocrinology, 107, 908–14
11. van Beurden, W. M. O., Roodnat, R. and van der Molen, H. J. (1978). Intern. J. Androl. Suppl., 2, 374–83
12. Hsueh, A. J. W., Dufau, M. L. and Catt, K. J. (1978). Endocrinology, 103, 1096–1102
13. Purvis, K. and Hansson, V. (1978). Mol. Cell. Endocrinol., 12, 123–38
14. Moger, W. H. and Murphy, P. R. (1982). Biol. Reprod., 26, 422–8
15. Hsueh, A. J. W. (1980). Biochem. Biophys. Res. Commun., 97, 506–12
16. Hsueh, A. J. W., Schreiber, J. R. and Frickson, G. F. (1981). Mol. Cell. Endocrinol., 21, 43–9
17. Verhoeven, G., Koninckx, P. and de Moor, P. (1982). J. Steroid Biochem., 17, 319–22
18. Mather, J. P., Saez, J. M. and Haour, F. (1981). Steroids, 38, 35–44
19. Mather, J. P., Saez, J. M. and Haour, F. (1982). Endocrinology, 110, 933–40
20. Haour, F., Dray, F. and Mather, J. P. (1982). Ann. N.Y. Acad. Sci., 383, 231–48
21. Saez, J. M., Benahmed, M., Reventos, J., Mombrial, F., Bommelaer, M. C. and Haour, F. (1983). J. Steroid Biochem., 19, 375–84
22. Benahmed, M., Bernier, M., Ducharme, J. R. and Saez, J. M. (1982). Mol. Cell. Endocrinol., December
23. Lefèvre, A., Saez, J. M. and Finaz, C. (1983). Horm. Res., 17, 114–20
24. Bohnet, H. G. and Friensen, H. G. (1976). J. Reprod. Fertil., 48, 307–11
25. Bex, F. J. and Bartke, A. (1977). Endocrinology, 100, 1223–6
26. Auclair, C., Kelly, P. A., Coy, D. H., Schally, A. V. and Labrie, F. (1977). Endocrinology, 101, 1890–3
27. Belanger, A., Auclair, C., Seguin, C., Kelly, P. A. and Labrie, F. (1979). Mol. Cell. Endocrinol., 13, 47–53
28. Sharpe, R. M. and McNeilly, A. S. (1979). Mol. Cell. Endocrinol., 18, 19–27
29. Purvis, K., Clausen, O. P. F., Olsen, A., Haug, E. and Hansson, V. (1979). Arch. Androl., 3, 219–30
30. Aragona, C., Bohnet, H. G. and Friesen, H. G. (1977). Acta Endocrinol. (Kbh), 84, 402–9
31. Aragona, C. and Friesen, H. H. (1975). Endocrinology, 97, 677–84
32. Freeman, D. A. and Ascoli, M. (1981). Proc. Natl. Acad. Sci. USA, 78, 6309–13
33. Dix, C. J. and Cooke, B. A. (1981). Biochem. J., 196, 713–19
34. Cusan, L., Belanger, A., Seguin, C. and Labrie, F. (1980). Mol. Cell. Endocrinol., 18, 165–76
35. Charreau, E. H., Calvo, J. C., Tesone, M., Biella de Souza, L. and Baranao, J. L. (1978). J. Biol. Chem., 253, 2504–6
36. Adashi, E. Y., Fabies, C. and Hsueh, A. J. W. (1982). Biol. Reprod., 26, 270–80
37. Haour, F. and Saez, J. M. (1978). In McKerns, K. W. (ed.) Structure and Function of the Gonadotropins. pp. 497–516. (New York: Plenum Press)

38. Nozu, K., Dehesia, A., Zawistowich, L., Catt, K. J. and Dufau, M. L. (1981). *J. Biol. Chem.*, **256**, 12875–82
39. Ascoli, M. (1982). *Ann. N.Y. Acad. Sci.*, **383**, 151–73
40. Huhtaniemi, I. T., Katikineni, M., Chan, V. and Catt, K. J. (1981). *Endocrinology*, **108**, 58–65
41. Hsueh, A. J. W., Dufau, M. L. and Catt, K. J. (1977). *Proc. Natl. Acad. Sci. USA*, **74**, 592–5
42. Saez, J. M., Haour, F. and Cathiard, A. M. (1978). *Biochem. Biophys. Res. Commun.*, **81**, 552–8
43. Ascoli, M. and Puett, D. (1978). *J. Biol. Chem.*, **253**, 4892–9
44. Rajaniemi, H. J., Mauninen, M. and Huhtaniemi, I. T. (1979). *Endocrinology*, **105**, 1208–14
45. Rajaniemi, H. J., Karjalainen, M., Veijola, M., *et al.* (1981). *J. Histochem. Cytochem.*, **29**, 813–20
46. Hsueh, A. J. W., Dufau, M. L., Katz, S. I. and Catt, K. J. (1977). *Nature (Lond.)*, **261**, 710–11
47. Begeot, M., Mombrial, F., Dubois, P. M., Dubois, M. P. and Haour, F. (1983). *J. Histochem. Cytochem.*, **31**, 898–904
48. Mombrial, C., Begeot, M., Leduque, P., Dubois, P., Saez, J. M. and Haour, F. (1984). *Biochem. Biophys. Res. Commun.*, **118**, 206–11
49. Auclair, C., Kelly, P. A., Labrie, F., Coy, D. H. and Schally, A. V. (1977). *Biochem. Biophys. Res. Commun.*, **76**, 855–62
50. Cusan, L., Auclair, C., Belanger, A., *et al.* (1979). *Endocrinology*, **104**, 1369–76
51. Hsueh, A. J. W. and Jones, P. B. C. (1981). *Endocr. Rev.*, **2**, 437–61
52. Arimura, A., Serafini, P., Talbot, S. and Schally, A. V. (1979). *Biochem. Biophys. Res. Commun.*, **90**, 687–93
53. Hsueh, A. J. W. and Erickson, G. F. (1979). *Nature (Lond.)*, **281**, 66–8
54. Hsueh, A. J. W. (1982). *Ann. N.Y. Acad. Sci.*, **383**, 249–72
55. Sharpe, R. M. and Cooper, I. (1982). *Mol. Cell. Endocrinol.*, **26**, 141–50
56. Sharpe, R. M., Doogan, D. G. and Cooper, I. (1982). *Biochem. Biophys. Res. Commun.*, **106**, 1210–17
57. Hunter, M. G., Sullivan, M. H. F., Dix, C. J., Aldred, L. F. and Cooke, B. A. (1982). *Mol. Cell. Endocrinol.*, **27**, 31–44
58. Sharpe, R. M. and Cooper, I. (1982). *Mol. Cell. Endocrinol.*, **27**, 199–211
59. Clayton, R. N. and Huhtaniemi, I. P. (1982). *Nature (Lond.)*, **299**, 56–9
60. Ascoli, M. (1982). (Discussion of paper 54)
61. Ascoli, M. (1981). *J. Biol. Chem.*, **256**, 179–83
62. Simpson, E. R. (1979). *Mol. Cell. Endocrinol.*, **13**, 213–27
63. Dufau, M. L. and Catt, K. J. (1978). *Vit. Horm.*, **36**, 461–592
64. Cooke, B. A., Lindh, L. M. and van der Molen, H. J. (1979). *Biochem. J.*, **184**, 33–8
65. Podesta, E. J., Dufau, M. L., Solano, A. R. and Catt, K. J. (1978). *J. Biol. Chem.*, **253**, 8994–9001
66. Lowit, S., Farese, R. V., Sabir, M. A. and Root, A. W. (1982). *Endocrinology*, **111**, 1415–17
67. van Beurden, M. O., Roodnat, B. and van der Molen, H. J. (1978). *Intern. J. Androl.* Suppl., **2**, 374–83
68. Savard, K., Marsh, J. M. and Rice, B. B. (1965). *Rec. Prog. Horm. Res.*, **21**, 285–365
69. Goldstein, J. L. and Brown, M. S. (1976). *Ann. Rev. Biochem.*, **48**, 897–930
70. Brown, M. S., Kovanen, P. T. and Goldstein, J. L. (1979). *Rec. Prog. Horm Res.*, **35**, 215–52
71. Carr, B. R. and Simpson, E. R. (1981). *Endocr. Rev.*, **2**, 306–26
72. Christie, M. H., Strauss, J. F. and Flickinger, G. L. (1979). *Endocrinology*, **105**, 92–8
73. Winkel, G. A., Snyder, J. M., MacDonald, P. C. and Simpson, E. R. (1980). *Endocrinology*, **106**, 1054–60
74. Morris, M. D. and Chaikoff, I. L. (1959). *J. Biol. Chem.*, **234**, 1045–97
75. Andersen, J. M. and Dietschy, J. M. (1978). *J. Biol. Chem.*, **253**, 9024–32
76. Chen, Y. D. I., Kraemer, F. B. and Reaven, G. M. (1980). *J. Biol. Chem.*, **255**, 9162–7
77. Schreiber, J. R., Weinstein, D. A. and Hsueh, A. J. W. (1982). *J. Steroid Biochem.*, **16**, 39–43
78. Benahmed, M., Dellamonica, C., Haour, F. and Saez, J. M. (1981). *Biochem. Biophys. Res. Commun.*, **99**, 1123–9
79. Murono, E. P. and Payne, A. H. (1979). *Biol. Reprod.*, **20**, 911–17
80. Hsueh, A. J. W., Schreiber, J. R. and Erickson, G. F. (1981). *Mol. Cell. Endocrinol.*, **21**, 43–9
81. Eik-Nes, K. (1971). *Rec. Progr. Horm. Res.*, **27**, 517–35
82. Cooke, B. A., Golding, M., Dix, C. J. and Hunter, M. G. (1982). *Mol. Cell. Endocrinol.*, **27**, 221–31
83. Zipf, W. P., Payne, A. H. and Kelch, R. P. (1978). *Biochim. Biophys. Acta*, **540**, 330–6
84. Saez, J. M., Haour, F., Tell, G. P., Gallet, D. and Sanchez, P. (1978). *Mol. Pharmacol.*, **14**, 1054–62
85. Jahnsen, T., Purvis, K., Torjensen, P. A. and Hansson, V. (1981). *Arch. Androl.*, **6**, 155–9

86. Dix, C. J. and Cooke, B. D. (1982). *Biochem. J.*, **204**, 613–16
87. Cigorraga, S. B., Dufau, M. L. and Catt, K. J. (1978). *J. Biol. Chem.*, **253**, 4297–4304
88. Saez, J. M., Morera, A. M. and Haour, F. (1979). In Dumont, J., Nunez, J. and van der Molen, H. J. (eds.) *Hormone and Cell Regulation.* Vol. 3, pp. 187–216. (Amsterdam: Elsevier-North Holland)
89. Chasalow, F., Marr, H., Haour, F. and Saez, J. M. (1978). *J. Biol. Chem.*, **253**, 5613–17
90. Brinkman, A. O., Leemborg, I., Rommerts, F. and van der Molen, H. J. (1982). *Endocrinology*, **110**, 1834–6
91. Dufau, M. L., Cigorraga, S., Baukal, A. J., *et al.* (1979). *Endocrinology*, **105**, 1314–21
92. Brinkman, A. O., Leemborg, F. G., Roodnat, E. M., de Jong, F. H. and van der Molen, H. J. (1980). *Biol. Reprod.*, **23**, 801–4
93. Garnier, F. and Saez, J. M. (1980). *Biol. Reprod.*, **22**, 832–6
94. Davies, T. F., Hodgen, C. D., Dufau, M. L. and Catt, K. J. (1979). *J. Clin. Invest.*, **64**, 1070–3
95. Saez, J. M. and Forest, M. G. (1979). *J. Clin. Endocrinol. Metab.*, **49**, 278–83
96. Forest, M. G., Lecoq, A. and Saez, J. M. (1979). *J. Clin. Endocrinol. Metab.*, **49**, 284–91
97. Benahmed, M., Reventos, J. and Saez, J. M. (1983). *Endocrinology*, **112**, 1952–7
98. Quinn, P. G., Dombrausky, L. J., Chen, Y. I. and Payne, A. H. (1981). *Endocrinology*, **109**, 1790–2
99. Kalla, N. R., Nisula, B. C., Menard, R. and Loriaux, D. L. (1980). *Endocrinology*, **106**, 35–9
100. Cigorraga, S. B., Sorrell, S., Bator, J., Catt, K. J. and Dufau, M. L. (1980). *J. Clin. Invest.*, **65**, 699–705
101. Moger, W. H. (1980). *Endocrinology*, **106**, 496–503
102. Nozu, K., Dufau, M. L. and Catt, K. J. (1981). *J. Biol. Chem.*, **256**, 1915–22
103. Brinkmann, A. O., Leemborg, F. G. and van der Molen, H. J. (1981). *Mol. Cell. Endocrinol.*, **24**, 65–72
104. Melner, M. H. and Abney, T. O. (1980). *Endocrinology*, **107**, 1620–6
105. Moger, W. H. (1980). *J. Steroid Biochem.*, **13**, 61–6
106. Brinkmann, A. O., Leemborg, F. G., Rommerts, F. F. G. and van der Molen, H. J. (1982). Presented at the *2nd European Workshop on Molecular and Cellular Endocrinology of the Testis*, Rotterdam, 1982, abstract B-5
107. Lipsett, M. B. (1980). *N. Engl. J. Med.*, **303**, 682–8
108. Rose, R. M., Gordon, T. P. and Berstein, I. S. (1972). *Science*, **178**, 643–5
109. Taché, Y., Ducharme, J. R., Charpenet, G., Haour, F., Saez, J. M. and Collu, R. (1980). *Acta Endocrinol.*, **93**, 168–74
110. Charpenet, G., Taché, Y., Forest, M. G., *et al.* (1981). *Endocrinology*, **109**, 1254–8
111. Doerr, P. and Pirke, K. M. (1976). *J. Clin. Endocrinol. Metab.*, **43**, 622–9
112. Saez, J. M., Morera, A. M., Haour, F. and Evain, D. (1979). *Endocrinology*, **101**, 1256–63
113. Bambino, T. H. and Hsueh, A. J. W. (1981). *Endocrinology*, **108**, 2142–8
114. Bernier, M., Gibb, W. and Ducharme, J. R. (1982). *Endocrinology*, Suppl. **110** (abstract 466)
115. Purvis, K., Clausen, O. P. F. and Hanssen, V. (1979). *Biol. Reprod.*, **20**, 304–9
116. Barney, K. J. and Ewing, L. (1981). *Endocrinology*, **109**, 993–5
117. Haour, F., Bommelaer, M. C., Sanchez, P., Saez, J. M. and Mather, J. P. (1983). *Mol. Cell. Endocrinol.*, **30**, 73–84
118. Adashi, E. Y. and Hsueh, A. J. W. (1981). *Nature (Lond.)*, **293**, 737–9
119. Hsueh, A. J. W., Welsh, T. H. and Jones, P. B. C. (1981). *Endocrinology*, **108**, 2002–4
120. Welsh, T. H. and Hsueh, A. J. W. (1982). *Endocrinology*, **110**, 1498–1506
121. Vaughan, M. K., Vaughan, G. M. and Klein, D. C. (1974). *Science*, **186**, 938–9
122. Yamashita, K., Mieno, M. and Yamashita, E. (1980). *J. Endocrinol.*, **84**, 449–52
123. Reiter, R. J. (1980). *Endocrinol. Rev.*, **1**, 109–38
124. Adashi, E. Y. and Hsueh, A. J. W. (1981). *Nature (Lond.)*, **293**, 650–2
125. Adashi, E. Y. and Hsueh, A. J. W. (1982). *J. Biol. Chem.*, **257**, 1301–8
126. de Kretser, D. M. (1982). *Int. J. Androl.*, Suppl. **5**, 11–17
127. Aoki, A. and Fawcett, D. W. (1978). *Biol. Reprod.*, **19**, 144–58
128. Risbridger, G. P., Kerr, J. B., Peake, R. A. and de Kretser, D. M. (1981). *Endocrinology*, **109**, 1234–41
129. Chubb, C. and Ewing, L. L. (1979). *Am. J. Physiol.*, **237**, E 247–E 254
130. Collu, R., Taché, Y. and Ducharme, J. R. (1982). *Endocrinology*, **110**, Suppl. Abstract 731
131. Ewing, L. L., Zirkin, B. R., Cochran, R. C., Kromann, N., Peters, C. and Ruiz-Bravo, N. (1979). *Endocrinology*, **105**, 1135–42
132. Zirkin, B. R., Ewing, L. L., Kromann, N. and Cochran, R. C. (1980). *Endocrinology*, **107**, 1867–74

III—Clinical Pathology

7
Evolution and function of non-ovulatory follicles

J. de Brux

INTRODUCTION

For many years, only the ovulatory follicle attracted the attention of histologists and physiologists, atretic follicles being considered as of no major interest. A continuation of this trend may be found today in the attention being paid to the 'dominant follicle', as a result of recent developments in the collection of mature oocytes by laparoscopy, *in vitro* fertilization and the success of ovum implantation at the earliest stage of development.

These many studies and important results have thus left in the shade those follicles which, although stimulated, never reach maturity but nevertheless exercise a specific influence on ovarian morphology, from the 24th week of intra-uterine life until the menopause. These non-ovulatory follicles also play a role in maintaining hormonal equilibrium from the first signs of puberty until well after the menopause.

In addition, menstrual cycle anomalies, as well as certain pathological states with a histogenesis that is still obscure, will be better understood after closer histological observation and a more thorough histochemical and histoenzymological analysis of atretic follicle constituents.

THE FOLLICLE IN FETAL LIFE AND INFANCY

The human follicle acquires its adult characteristics during the last months of intra-uterine life, infancy and pre-puberty. During this period, the full complement of fetal primordial follicles reaches completion, and differentiation of tissue constituents occurs.

The nature and kinetics of the complex ovarian structures were first observed and described by de Graaf in 1672 and, nearly three centuries later, by Hill and White in 1933[1].

By approximately 7–8 months of intra-uterine life, the number of follicles can be as high as 6 million, but it regresses rapidly.

From the 32nd week, the prenatal ovary, as well as that of the new-born child, is composed of oocytes surrounded by one or two granulosa precursory cells with a peripheral connective reticulum containing fibroblasts, smooth muscle cells and capillaries (Figure 1). The origin of functional ovarian cells is controversial: some embryologists believe that cords of granulosa cells that surround the gonocytes and penetrate with them originate from the coelomic mesothelium covering the gonadal anlage[2-6]. Five such surges of oocytes may occur.

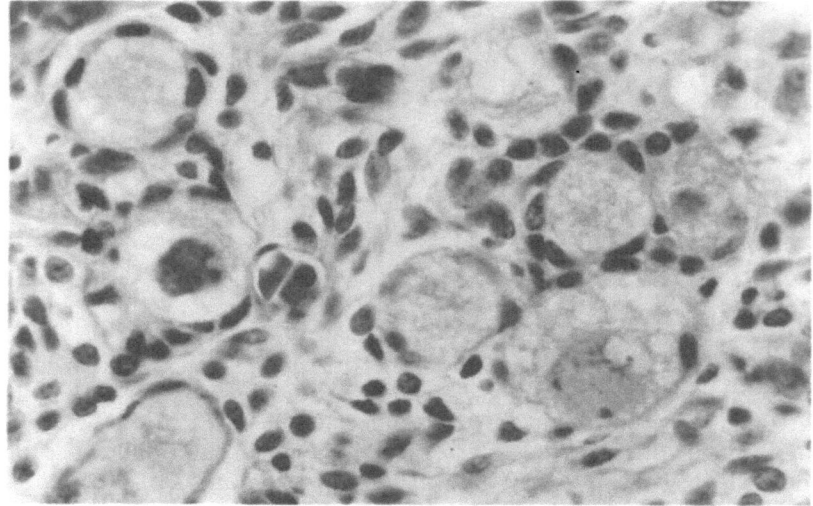

Figure 1 Ovarian follicles of an 8-month fetus. The granulosa cells are well developed round the oocytes. Numerous elongated cells and capillaries surround the granulosa cells (× 560)

Others[7,8] believe that the gonocytes are surrounded by the mesenchyme cells of the genital crest arising from coelomic mesothelium. Moreover, Gruenwald[9] and Torrey[10] believe that surface mesothelial cells are also involved.

For Merchant[11] the cells of the mesonephros are active in the formation of the ovary.

According to Waldeyer[12], Witschi[13] and Mauleon[14] two surges occur in the formation of the ovary:

(1) That of the surface mesothelial cells.
(2) That of the vestiges of the mesonephros (rete ovarii), their vessels penetrating into the developing ovary after regression of the medulla.

These considerations are of practical as well as of scientific interest, as they could explain the special sensitivity to FSH of the granulosa cells in direct contact with the oocyte, whereas the internal theca cells respond essentially to LH: the respective receptors to these protein hormones and their enzyme responses are therefore different, probably because of their *different embryonic origin*.

Before and after birth, a great number of oogonia and oocytes become atretic, and primordial follicles are distributed over the entire surface of the gonad. A few follicles with a cavity in the process of atresia persist in the medulla, but the majority are situated on the superficial part of the cortex and some may still form even 4 months after birth. After a few months of extra-uterine life, all follicles are limited to this zone.

Follicular growth begins in the fetus and neonate. Certain follicles begin to grow, then degenerate; this activity is particularly notable during the first 4 months of life, when FSH and LH levels are high. The ovaries of children dying from trauma between the ages of 2 months and 11 years even show the presence of pre-antral follicles. After the age of 6, antral follicles are found to increase in number with the child's age. Scars of old follicles are also seen, indicating that they have undergone a process of evolution followed by regression. The internal theca surrounding the follicles is thickened, which is a sign of FSH and LH stimulation inducing follicle growth during the first years of life.

In the child, as in the rat, but less distinctly, follicle growth occurs in three phases:

(1) *An infantile phase*, during which the ovary does not respond to gonado-trophins.
(2) *An early phase*, in which steroidogenesis appears after gonadotrophin stimu-lation (enzyme development, with a steroidogenic response to FSH/LH and PGE_2, probably begins in the early stage).
(3) *A late phase*, terminating in the growth and maturation of the follicle.

STIMULATED FOLLICLES

Primordial follicles are formed of a basal membrane, granulosa cells and one oocyte (sometimes, but rarely, two oocytes, except in amenorrhoeic patients receiving gonadotrophins to stimulate follicle growth) (Figure 2). They are situated near the albuginea, whereas cystic follicles are distributed within the

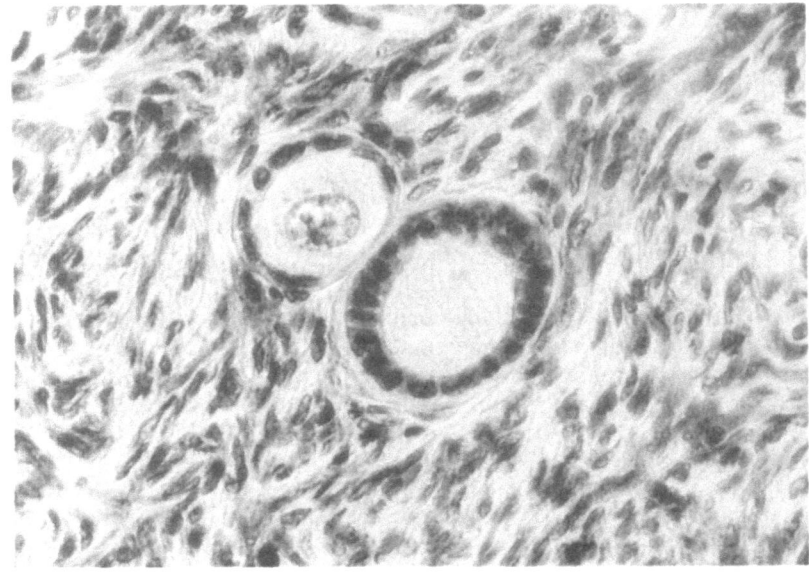

Figure 2 Primordial follicle and developing follicle with multiplication of granulosa cells (× 480)

97

cortex. Follicle growth is continuous throughout every cycle, pregnancy and even under oral contraception, especially when this is given in minute doses.

Oocyte development and *granulosa cell* multiplication mark the beginning of the growth of the follicle, which penetrates into the stroma as it develops.

The flattened stroma cells at the exterior of the basement membrane become vascularized and are later transformed into the *internal theca cells* (Figure 3). This layer is composed of fibroblastic and smooth muscle cells (their existence is questioned by Reeves[15], although the presence of antimyosin antibodies has been demonstrated). Glycogen, lipids and the enzymes necessary for steroidogenesis are present in the granulosa and theca cells. However, the *different embryonic origin* of *granulosa and theca cells* is shown by alterations in the nature of the granulosa cell esterases after luteinization.

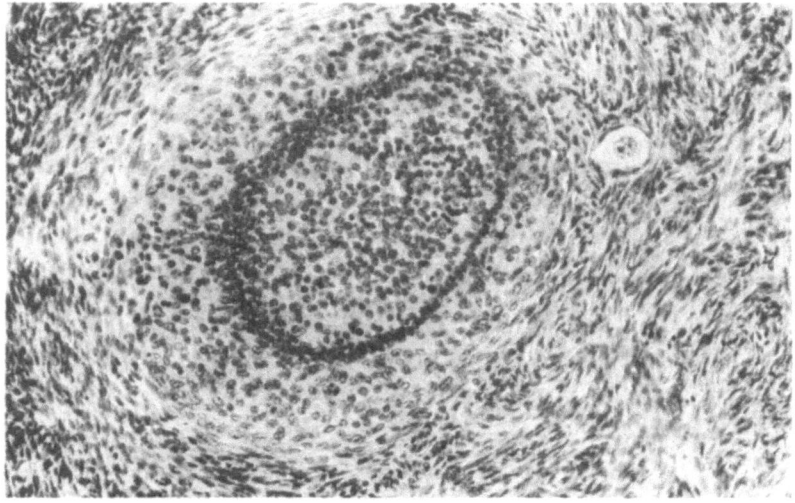

Figure 3   Pre-antral follicle (200 μm) showing theca cell differentiation   (× 140)

Granulosa cells

Granulosa cells, which are flattened in primordial follicles, become cuboid at the time of growth and division, then round out and form concentric layers around the oocyte.

Anderson[16] described very small canaliculi communicating the periphery of the follicle with the surrounding medium. The oocyte itself is also in contact with this medium via the spaces that appear in contact with the oocyte. At the beginning of development, the granulosa cells are mutually coherent, maintaining a specific environment around the oocyte; gradually, as growth progresses, fissures between adjacent granulosa cells widen and permit communication and exchange between the cells. Furthermore, these gaps ('Call–Exner bodies') facilitate rapid cell response to hormones. Microvillosities appear at the surface of the granulosa cells of the medium-sized follicles, and are evidence of the response to gonadotrophins. From this moment on, these cells possess LH receptors, as these villosities will disappear on the formation of the corpus luteum.

Granulosa cells multiply rapidly during the periods of follicle growth. They secrete the follicular fluid which accumulates to form the antrum and push the oocyte and its cumulus proliger to one side of the follicle (Figure 4). At the moment of ovulation, these cells secrete large quantities of glycoaminoglycans, whereas the cells near the basement membrane are richer in gonadotrophin receptors. The number of layers of granulosa cells and the size of the antrum are a basis for the classification of the stages of follicle growth.

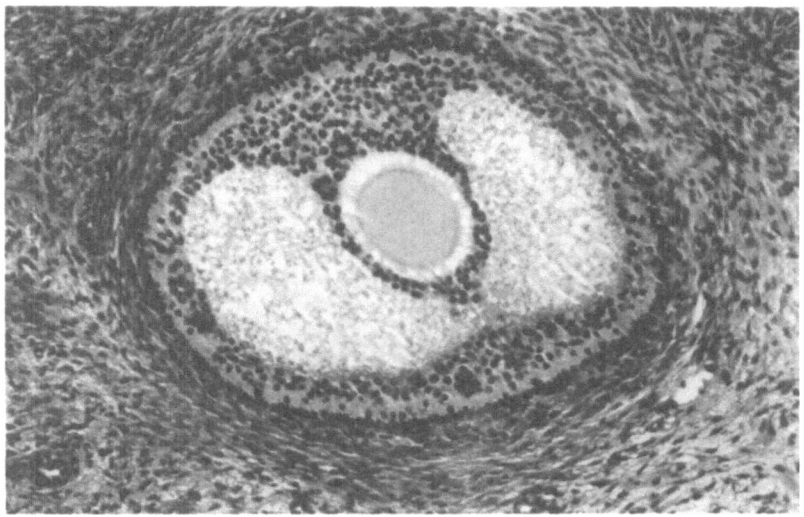

Figure 4   Small antral follicle   ($\times$ 300)

Thecal cells

Similarly, the importance of theca cells and their relationship to granulosa cells has, until now, been insufficiently understood and appreciated. The basement membrane is not a frontier, but a zone of *exchange*.

Theca cells become differentiated when the pre-antral follicle attains an approximate diameter of 200 μm: granulosa cells play a role in their differentiation. Chemically, the theca is characterized by the presence of cells loaded with lipid that becomes transformed into steroids; these cells also synthesize glycoaminoglycans and regulate the oocyte. But inversely, the oocyte may act upon follicle growth. Thus in the 'resistant ovary syndrome', the following situation may occur: the follicles are intact, but are incapable of growing. This incapacity may be related either to the impossibility of granulosa cells organizing the follicle, or to oocyte insufficiency.

REGULATION OF GROWTH

During each menstrual cycle, approximately 50 follicles grow enough to reach 1 mm in diameter. But of these only three at most reach 8 mm at mid-cycle. A mature follicle is about 2–3 cm in diameter.

Follicle development and early growth regulation is established by an amazingly regular and well-ordered control system. At its beginning, growth is not dependent on pituitary hormones, but is autonomous and, even after hypophysectomy, continues up to the antral stage. Regulating factors may be follicle number, subject age and perhaps also inhibitory substances in the follicular liquid of larger follicles. This growth begins in a specific order, perhaps in the same order as follicle formation in the fetal ovary, a hypothesis known as the 'first in, first out' theory. (This would explain why, in the neonate, stimulated follicles are found in the deep part of the ovary.)

Pedersen[17] calls 'transit time' the interval during which a follicle passes from one stage to the next. The duration of the follicular growth period covers several cycles. In the rat, 5 weeks are necessary for a follicle with a single layer of cuboid cells to become a Graafian follicle; in women, this transformation takes 60–90 days.

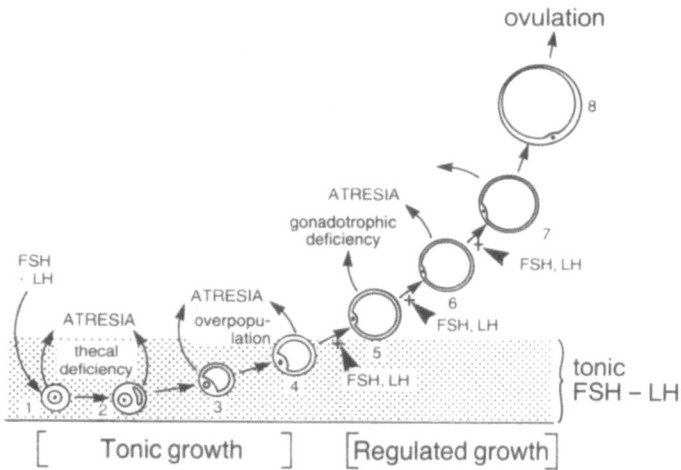

Figure 5 Tonic and regulated follicular growth and involution. The shadow area represents the tonic secretion of LH and FSH. This secretion assumes the growth of the follicles from the type 1 to 4. The atresia of these types is essentially linked to the inadequate differentiation of the internal theca or to a surpopulation (type 3 and 4). A gonadotrophic supplementary secretion is needed from the following development of the follicle types 5, 6 and 7. A hormonal deficiency related to the gonadotrophic pulses induces the atresia of some of them (From Gougeon, A. (1981). Thesis, University of Paris)

Gonadotrophin action is essential in the final stages leading to maturation, and this action is marked by two periods (Figure 5):

(1) A *tonic* period, during which the rate of gonadotrophin secretion is sufficient to ensure follicle growth from type 1 to type 4. Atresia at this point can be due either to inadequate internal theca differentiation (types 1 and 2), or to overpopulation (types 3 and 4).

(2) A *regulated* period is characterized by a supplementary increase in gonadotrophin secretion, which is necessary for follicle development from type 5 to type 7 (Figure 6) (whence the interest of the 'LH-pump' to induce

complete follicle maturation). Nevertheless, most follicles become atretic, due to cyclical gonadotrophin fluctuation or to possible FSH–LH receptors insufficiencies[18,19].

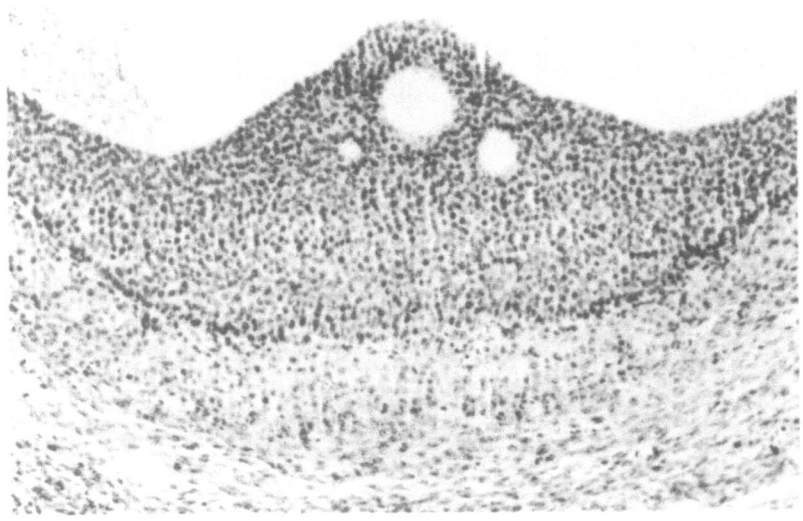

Figure 6 Follicle types 7 and 8 (× 120)

FOLLICULAR ATRESIA

Growing follicles may be classified into different types according to size; various aetiologies lie behind atresia, and it is associated with special endocrine phenomena.

Atresia occurs at all stages of the follicular cycle (Figure 7). In the neonate and child, all follicles that begin to grow degenerate. At the onset of puberty, about 10 follicles reach type 6–7 of the antral stage, but atresia appears as the antrum widens, and becomes total between types 6 and 8 (1000–6000 μm). Around puberty and the menopause, large follicles may become cystic if gonadotrophin stimulation is insufficient, poorly received or unbalanced. These cysts are thus frequent with strong and permanent E_2 stimulation, blocking the LH peak, as is seen frequently in post-puberty and peri-menopause.

Atresia of primordial and primary follicles

Granulosa cells are progressively crushed, encompassed by hyaline sclerosis, whereas the oocyte becomes pyknotic and disappears (Figure 8).

Atresia of pre-antral follicles (class 1)

The granulosa cells are now all pyknotic and necrotic. In contrast, the internal theca appears still flourishing and even thickened. Geugeon[20] considers that this is only apparent, and due simply to follicle retraction. We, on the other hand, believe that the theca cells have enough gonadotrophin receptors to allow normal growth (Figure 9).

101

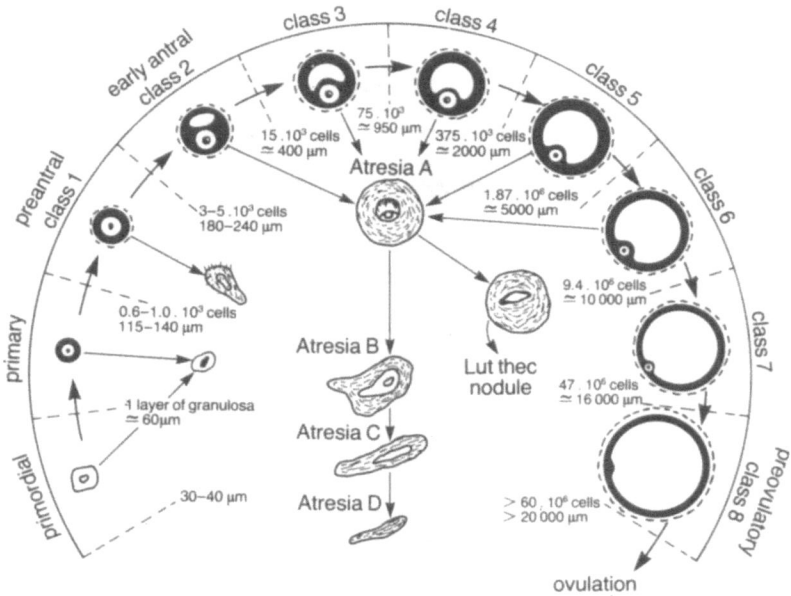

Figure 7 Atresia of different follicle types (Adapted from Peters, *et al.* (1978). *Clin. Endocrinol. Metab.*, 7, 469; and Gougeon (1981). PhD Thesis, University of Paris)

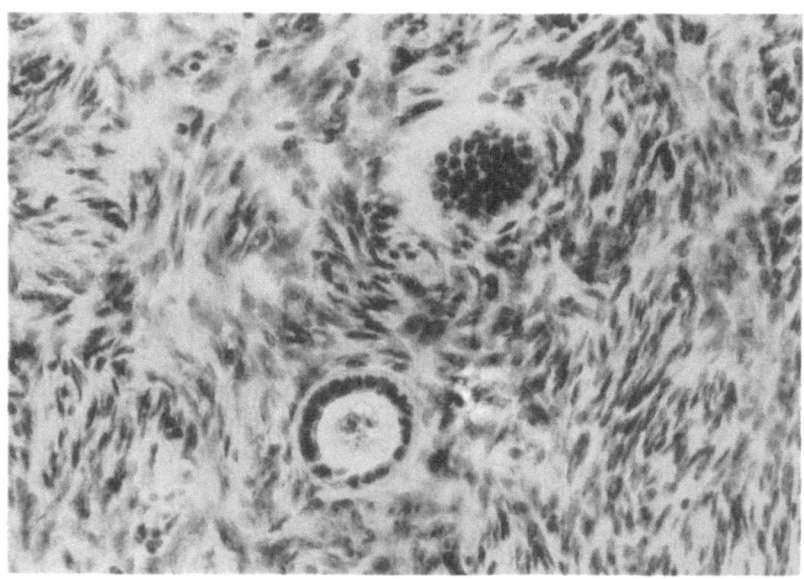

Figure 8 Pre-antral follicle with crushed granulosa cells, vanished oocytes and early sclerosis (× 480)

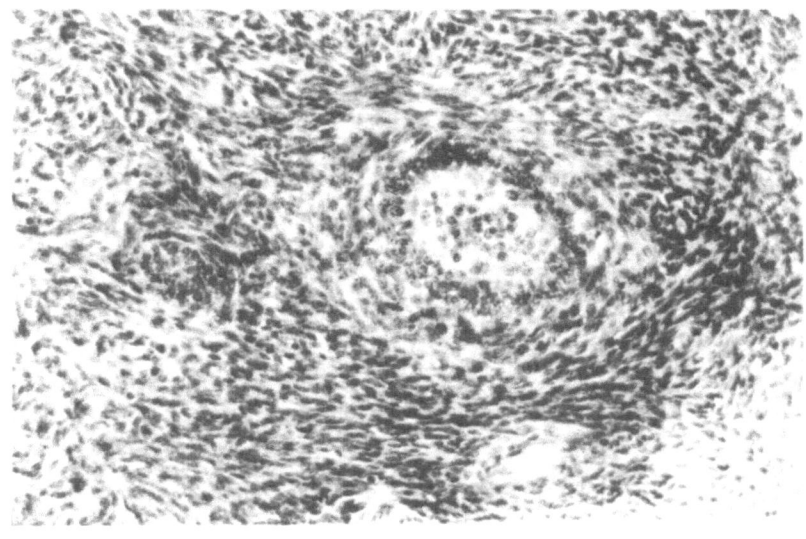

Figure 9 Atresia of follicle types 4 and 5 (× 300)

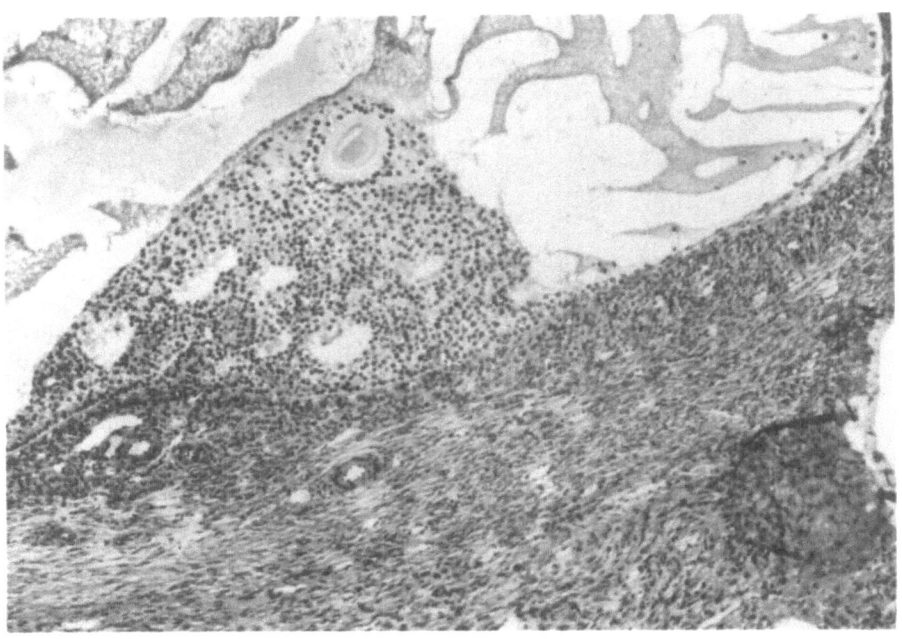

Figure 10 Atresia A. The cumulus proliger becomes smooth. The oocyte empties, and follicular fluid becomes denser (× 140)

103

Antral follicle atresia (class 2–5)

The involution period is very long and ends with follicle integration with the stroma. Several stages may be distinguished in this process:

Atresia A—The state of the oocyte nucleus is sometimes difficult to determine: the nucleolus may be transparent, the chromatin dispersed or the nucleus itself may lie at the periphery. The granulosa cells are morphologically normal (Figure 10).

Atresia B—The follicle is ovoid in form and, on one-quarter of its periphery, the granulosa has disappeared. The oocyte nucleus is pushed back, cumulus cells scatter, the basement membrane thickens and the internal theca cells atrophy (Figure 11).

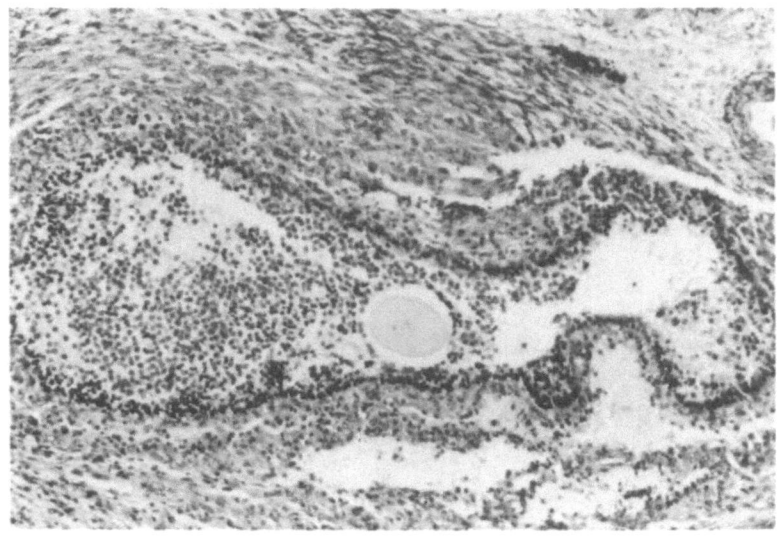

Figure 11   Atresia B   (× 120)

Atresia C—The follicle is irregular in form. The granulosa has disappeared; the oocyte, which is in the process of being resorbed, may persist, floating on the liquid, while the internal theca becomes the 'interstitial gland' (Figure 12).

Atresia D—The follicle is variable in form. The antrum shrinks and becomes invaded by connective tissue. The Slavjanski membrane is very thick, and hyalinized. The internal theca cells dedifferentiate and are integrated in their turn into the stroma (Figure 13)

The process of regression could be related to inadequate differentiation of the internal theca cells, which are LH dependent. If such is the case, then perhaps the internal theca of the follicles that have undergone early differentiation is more likely to avoid atresia; similarly, other follicles may regress because of inadequate gonadotrophin levels, or because their internal theca has imperfectly differentiated, with insufficient receptors.

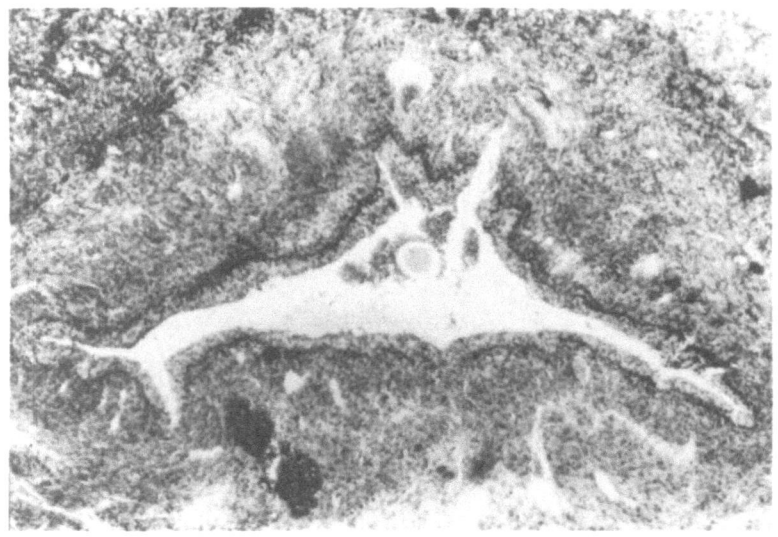

Figure 12 Atresia C (× 120)

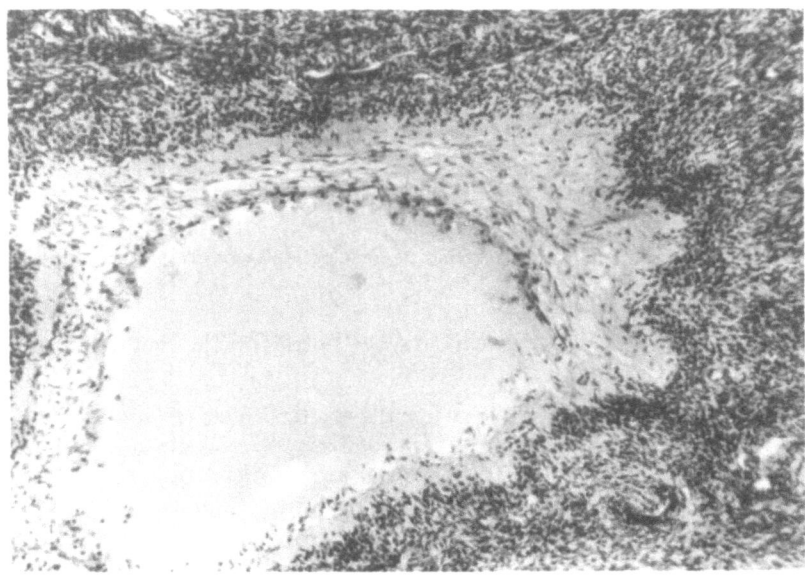

Figure 13 Atresia D (× 120)

In some cases, on the contrary, LH predominance leads to proliferation and especially to thecal luteinization (Figure 14).

These histological occurrences, already minutely described by Dubreuilh in 1935[21,22] are frequently found in the ovaries of women with menstrual disorders or simple or adenomatous endometrial hyperplasia, uterine leiomyomas or polycystic ovaries. These changes in the ovary may or may not enter into the definition of polycystic and/or Stein–Leventhal ovaries. In any case, in the ovaries of most of these patients there does exist some hyperplasia of the internal theca, which shows cytological signs of functional activity, often with high plasma E_2 levels.

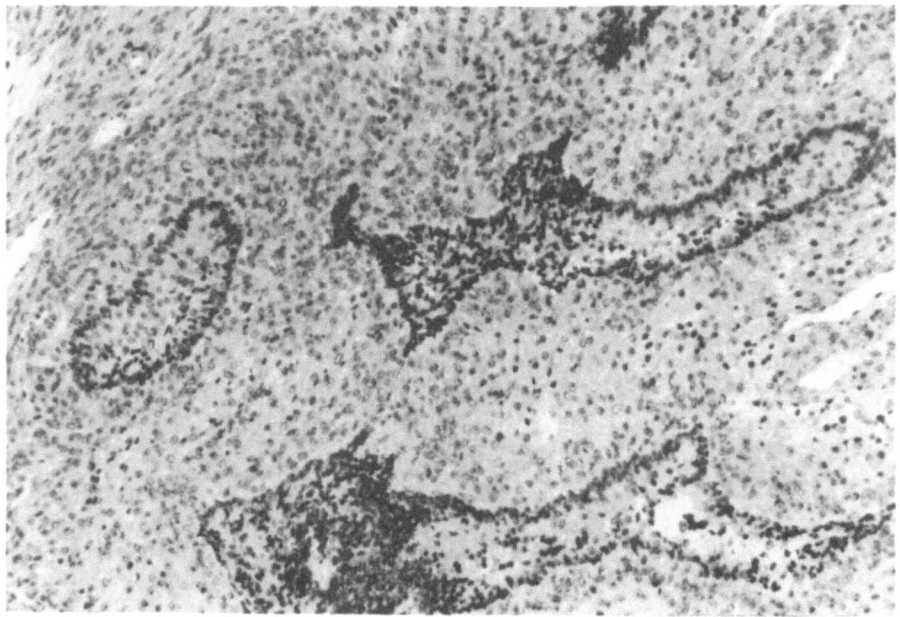

Figure 14 Theca cell proliferation surrounding granulosa cells with crushed antrum ($\times$ 350)

Internal theca hyperplasia appears in type 2 antral follicles, but mainly in those of types 3 and 4. There are two varieties:

(1) The more frequent variety is when the atretic follicle resembles a follicle in the course of development, except that the oocyte is degenerating. In this group, the granulosa cell layers are often disintegrating, but the internal theca remains active and thick, with polyhedral cells rich in lipids (Figure 15).

(2) In the second variety, mitoses are very common and the cells, which are polyhedral, eosinophilic and rich in lipids, are 'luteinized'. They can undergo intense proliferation and fill the antrum, pushing back and then replacing the few remaining granulosa cells (Figure 16). This is the appearance that Dubreuilh[21,22] described under the term of 'interstitial gland of the ovary'.

After several cycles, these 'luteinized thecal nodules' slowly become integrated into the stroma. The thecal cells stretch out, gradually lose their secretory character and contract, .often leaving a cell nodule made up of whorled and elongated cells. They nevertheless retain a steroidogenic potential and are still coloured by lipid stains. These thecal nodules are found especially in the ovaries of women exposed to high, and particularly to unbalanced gonadotrophin levels, as in the Stein–Leventhal syndrome. These formations should not be confused

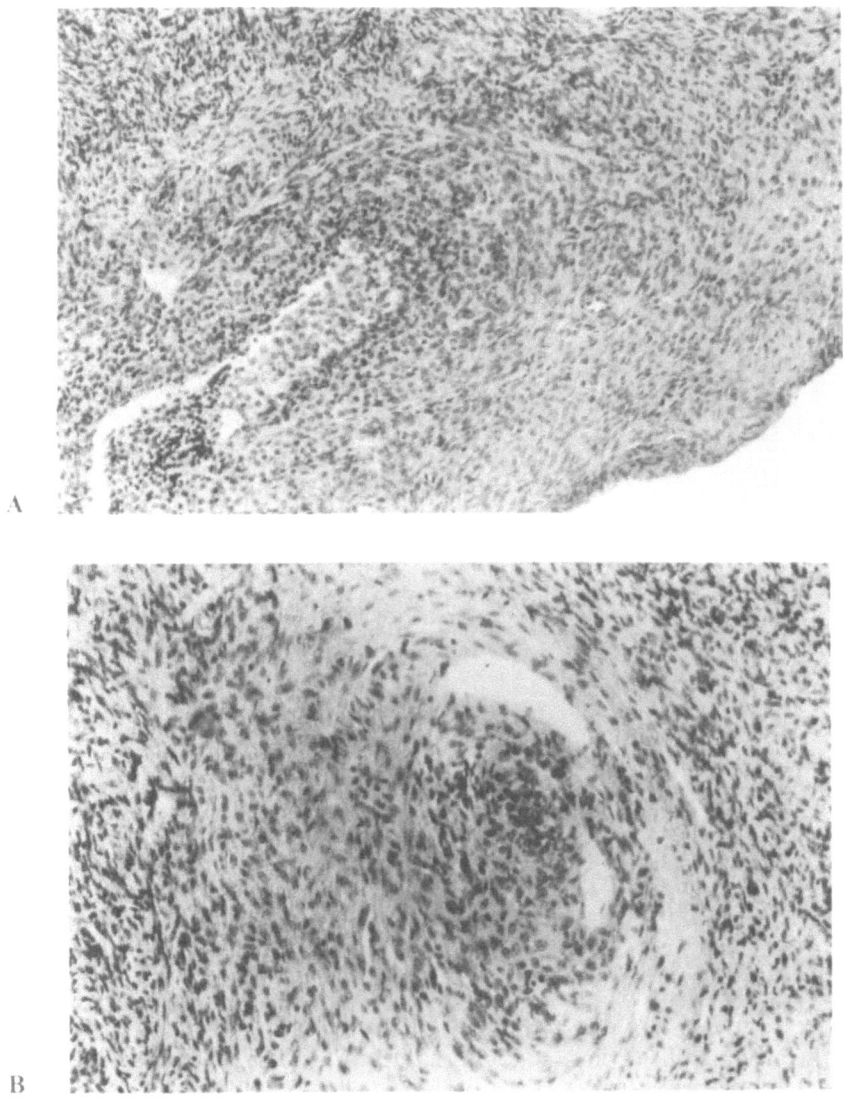

Figure 15 Theca cell proliferation pushing back and obliterating the antrum (A × 140; B × 300)

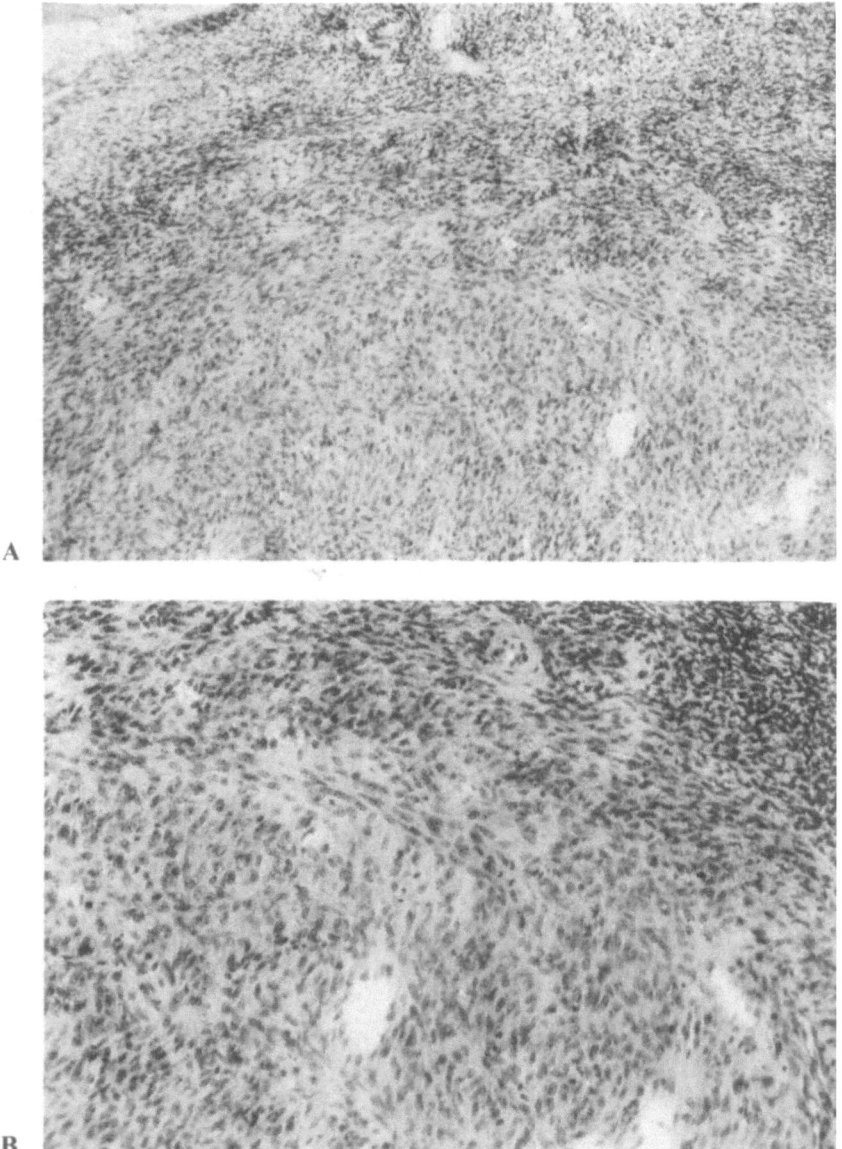

Figure 16 Dubreuilh's interstitial nodule. Multiplication of theca cells, which preserve their secretory features   (A × 120; B × 300)

with the atretic follicles close to corpora lutea in ovaries that have been hyper-stimulated by hCG (Figure 17).

Excessive proliferation is called by some authors 'hyperthecosis' or simply 'thecosis'. This entity (which Feinberg [23] divides into 'internal thecosis' and 'combined thecosis', i.e. associated or not with the presence of numerous follicular cysts) is a sign of disturbance in the balance of the gonadotrophins, particularly in their receptors in the granulosa and internal theca cells. This stromal proliferation (which may show functional activity at any stage in active genital life, but also in the peri- and post-menopause) occurs most often in women with high gonadotrophin levels and a high number of follicular receptors, but with a predominance of LH receptors on internal theca cells.

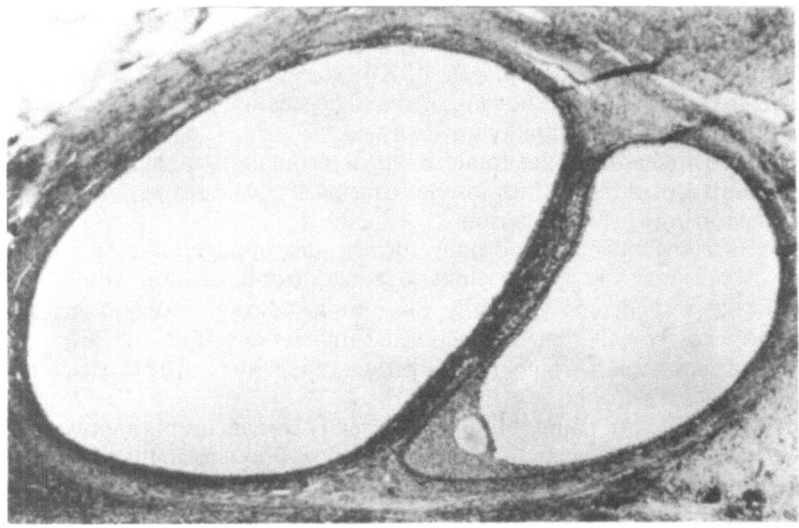

Figure 17   Pre-ovulatory follicle atresia in the PCO syndrome   (× 48)

These findings are confirmed by Richards[19], who considers that disturbances in theca cell FSH and LH receptor distribution bring about a degree of thecal hyperplasia and function. Furthermore, in some cases, persistence of FSH receptors leads at the same time to excessive theca cell proliferation, probably by stimulating the oxidizing enzymes of glucose 6-phosphatase dehydrogenase (G-6 PD) and 3β-hydroxysteroid dehydrogenase (3βOHSD). Abnormal aromatization of theca cell secretion is the cause of high androstenedione levels, as occurs in some cases of the Stein–Leventhal syndrome.

Pre-ovulatory follicles (classes 6, 7 and 8)

The atresia of these follicles is regulated by intra-follicular protein factors, but particularly by extra-ovarian factors (FSH, LH, prolactin) and intra-ovarian factors (oestradiol-17β, progesterone, prostaglandins, androstenedione). Their roles are not yet fully understood and are often contradictory[24].

A decrease in FSH or an imbalance in the FSH/LH ratio may have an atretic effect on the follicle by causing degeneration of the oocyte (lipid accumulation, formation of the pro-nucleus, or sometimes fragmentation). For Dyskov[25] oocytes are the first to be affected, whereas granulosa cells remain flourishing for longer.

Oestrogens, androgens that are aromatizable into oestrogens, and progesterone have an anti-atretic action on the follicle, although in very high levels this action is reversed, probably through inhibition of the releasing hormones and gonadotrophins.

Causes and consequences of the first stages of atresia

Normal development of the ovary is halted in some hereditary conditions, or in embryonic gonadal disorders. In these cases, 'streak ovaries' are found, with changes in the genital apparatus at birth and primary amenorrhoea at puberty. These disorders include various intersexual states, certain forms of ovarian dysgenesis and chromosomal anomalies.

The most widely known form is the 45 X0 streak ovary, manifested by abnormal ovarian growth, the gonad showing scattered degenerate germinal cells or primordial follicles that regress rapidly once formed.

The same appearances are found in chromosomal anomalies: deletion of the long or short arm of the X-chromosome, causing 45 X0/46 XX gonadal dysgenesis, with amenorrhoea, 18 or 21 trisomy.

At puberty, the follicles are normally formed; they appear numerous and normal on ovarian biopsy but are resistant to gonadotrophin action, resulting in the resistant ovary syndrome. Clinically, this is an instance of primary amenorrhoea; ovarian biopsy reveals that the primordial follicles have failed to grow; plasma gonadotrophin levels are high, and E_2 production is small, despite stimulation by exogenous gonadotrophins.

Possible causes are many, but none are really convincing: immunity, gonadotrophin receptor insufficiency, absence of granulosa/theca cell induction, hereditary disorders, etc.

The *insensitive ovary* is a similar disorder and occurs in women who have been treated with the combined contraceptive pill over a long period.

The *de Morsier–Kalman* syndrome (or olfacto-genital syndrome) is amenorrhoea caused by gonadotrophin and oestrogen insufficiency. However, the lesion here is hypothalamo-hypophyseal rather than ovarian, since administration of exogenous gonadotrophins induces ovulation.

Causes and functional activity of classes 2–5 atretic follicles

Functional activity seems to exist only in the internal theca of regressing follicles. Granulosa cells undergo lysis during follicle disintegration, but some steroids persist in the follicular fluid, together with FSH, LH, PG_2 and particularly protein factors such as inhibin, which plays a part in the determination of the ovulatory follicle.

Insufficient LH compared with FSH and FSH/LH receptor imbalance in the follicular cells lead to distension and hypotrophy of the internal theca, creating cystic follicles.

However, we have paid more particular attention to the role of thecal hyperplasia in the histogenesis of stromal hyperplasia in adult and peri-menopausal women, as well as of certain dystrophic and polycystic ovarian syndromes.

The terms 'stromal hyperplasia' and 'hyperthecosis' are considered as synonymous by some authors, whereas others assign them separate meanings. Nevertheless, Roddick and Greene[26] defined ovarian thecosis as an entity that includes the internal theca of a number of cystic follicles and also the cells of the cortical stroma. Feinberg[22] divides 'ovarian thecosis' into:

Sub-group 1, or 'internal thecosis'—Characterized by ovaries with follicular cysts, collagenization of the albuginea and predominance of normal or altered theca cells, but without any cortical stroma cells. The Stein–Leventhal syndrome belongs to this group.

Sub-group 2, or 'combined thecosis'—In which many follicular cysts are found, with thickening of the albuginea, and cortical stroma cells that are not derived from the internal theca.

The granulosa cells of these first two groups are not functional and are most often atrophic or lysed.

Sub-group 3, or 'cortical stroma thecosis'—Without follicles, is characterized by scattering of the stromal cells and is found in menopausal women. This group includes the stroma of primitive ovarian tumours and metastases.

In reality, these distinctions would seem rather tenuous, and we prefer the definition of Roddick and Greene[26].

Causes and consequences of classes 6–8 non-ovulatory follicles

Disorders of follicles belonging to classes 6–8 are defined by anovulation.

Histologically, they are characterized by non-rupture immaturity. The granulosa cells of many follicles are prematurely luteinized; conversely, other follicles are cystic without having been luteinized. But even after normal ovulation, functional disorders are frequent: long or short follicular or luteal phases.

All these disturbances induce infertility, endometrial hyperplasia and menstrual disorders. These disorders are essentially under the dependence of the gonadotrophins, acting on follicular secretion, and of intrafollicular factors.

Table 1 *Primordial follicles. N^1:* oocyte surrounded by one layer of flat cells

Histology	Clinical syndrome	Pathogenesis
Atresia: —nuclear piknosis —cytoplasmic eosinophilia —perifollicular sclerosis	Sexual and somatic anomalies	Genetic errors: XO, mosaics, ...
	Olfactogenital syndrome (Kallman, de Morsier)	Hypothalamic lesions
	Precocious menopause	Oocytic defects
	Resistant ovary syndrome	Granulosa cell inability to grow and organize the follicle

Table 2 *Primary and pre-antral follicles. Normal:* oocyte enlargement; granulosa cell proliferation; zona pellucida

Histology	Clinical syndrome	Pathogenesis
Atresia: —nuclear piknosis —cytoplasmic eosinophilia —granulosa cell degeneration —phagocytosis		Errors of meiosis
		Metabolic disorders
		Oocyte degeneration through penetration of hilar mesonephrotic cells
Integration into the stroma		FSH and LH receptor disorders

Table 3 *Antral follicles (classes 2, 3, 4, 5). Normal:* GN dependency; antrum with well differentiated granulosa and thecal cells; Slavjanski membrane

Histology	Clinical syndrome	Pathogenesis
(1) Oocyte disappearance: —crushed granulosa cells —penetration into antrum	Blunting of E_2 or Δ_4 secretion Pg insufficiency	FSH/LH receptor disorders in the follicular cells FSH/LH disorders
(2) Luteinization of granulosa cells Trapped oocyte Accessory C.L. of Weir and Rowlans		

Table 4 *Graafian follicle (classes 6 and 7).* GN dependency

Histology	Clinical syndrome	Pathogenesis
(1) Polycystic ovary: —multiple cysts layered by degenerated granulosa or theca cells —stromal hyperplasia	Oligo- or amenorrhoea through E_2 deficiency	A combination of causes: Androg. secretion by small cysts Low E_2 inducing permanent FSH with low and irregular LH
(2) Stein–Leventhal cysts with luteinized hyper-plastic cells Stromal hyperplasia	Oligo- or amenorrhoea A.H.T. hirsutism Large white ovaries	Low E_2 inducing persistent middle of the range FSH and LH levels without an ovulatory peak Adrenal stimulation→Androg. → E_2 Granulosa/theca cell imbalance follicular atresia Hypothalamic disorders (?)

Table 5 *Ovulatory follicle (class 8).* 1 cycle in 10 is anovulatory

Histology	Clinical syndrome	Pathogenesis
No ruptured follicle (trapped oocyte)	Infertility Stigma absent Enlarged ovary Pain Oedema	LH high but insufficient and/or precocious Intrafollicular factors HCG high or LH high Permanent FSH
Premature luteinization of many follicles, but no luteinization and some cysts formation in others	Endometrial hyperplasia Haemorrhage	E_2 Absent LH
Luteinization: Follicular phase long / short Luteal phase short or disturbed	Long cycle Short cycles (menopause) Oligomenorrhoea Infertility	FSH/LH imbalance Luteolysis Prolactin Vascular insufficiency Immunological (endometriosis) and inflammatory causes

DISCUSSION

Embryologically, part of the ovarian mesenchyma arises from the medulla and mesonephros, i.e. from the embryonic mesoblast which has first formed the mesonephros and then the genital crest; the gonocytes have penetrated into this preliminary anlage, bringing with them the cells of the surface mesothelium which, classically, are the precursors of the granulosa: these are the sex cords. The theca cells are very probably of mesonephrotic origin and their morphological and functional differentiation is induced by the oocyte and the granulosa cells, and also by gonadotrophin stimulation which regulates their multiplication and functional differentiation. Secondarily, these cells become integrated into the stroma.

At puberty, gonadotrophin action is focused on a group of follicles. The perifollicular cells respond to cyclical FSH/LH stimulation and, once this stimulation is exhausted, they return to a quiescent phase, increasing the amount of stroma in proportion to the degree of cell response to gonadotrophin stimulation. However, 'quiescence' does not mean that these cells are not able to respond again to high gonadotrophin stimulation, which is all the stronger for not having been braked by E_2 and P negative feedback, as is the case in the menopause.

This hypothesis is borne out by the biochemical and enzyme data, which show the narrow margin separating the ovarian tissue activity of women with a normal cycle from those with the disorders seen in various anatomoclinical syndromes. This emphasizes the cellular *plasticity* of all the components of the genital apparatus: differentiation, dedifferentiation, re-differentiation—so frequent in neoplasia, in the ovary they are manifested more by function than morphology in the different periods of life.

CONCLUSION

The ovary, which starts life at the 24th week of gestation, does not end its life until a long time after depletion of its follicular capital. All its constituent elements play an important functional role. During embryonic and early fetal life, the germinal cells act upon the surrounding mesenchymal cells. They thus preserve their embryonic and functional potential and are able to respond to gonadotrophin stimulation and to synthesize steroids and protein hormones.

From the 6th year onwards, the primordial follicles respond increasingly to pituitary stimulation. Multiplying follicular cells are integrated into the stroma, which thickens. The process is regulated during puberty with the beginning of regular menstrual cycles and ovulation.

Until the present day, non-ovulatory follicular atresia had been neither well classified nor timed.

The appearances observed in the ovaries are better understood today, thanks to a combination of the different approaches—histological, endocrinological and clinical. Correlation with the clinical findings can now be made, particularly where the integration into the stroma of hyperplastic, luteinized theca cells is concerned.

Oestrogen and/or androsterone secretion by these cells maintains for a long time a minimal steroid level after follicular depletion. Moreover, these cells are capable of returning to functional activity, with excessive or abnormal secretion in some pathological cases. This demonstrates the extraordinary plasticity of the gonadal cells and their ability to respond to gonadotrophin stimulation and also, on occasion, to assume their independence.

References

1. Hill, M. and White, W. E. (1933). The growth and regression of follicles in oestrous rabbit. *J. Physiol.*, **80**, 174
2. Baker, T. B. (1971). Gamatogenesis. In Proceedings of the *Symposium on the Use of Non-primates for Research on Problems of Human Reproduction*, p. 18
3. Carlon, N. and Stahl, A. (1973). Les premiers stades du développement des gonades chez l'homme et les vertébrés supérieurs. *Pathol. Biol.*, **21**, 903
4. Langman (1981). *Abrégé d'Embryologie Médicale*, 2nd edn. (Paris: Masson)
5. Moore, K. L. (1977). *The Developing Human. Clinically Oriented Embryology*. (Philadelphia: W. B. Saunders)
6. Tuchman-Duplessis, H. and Haegel, P. (1970). *Embryologie Humaine Illustrée*. T.2. (Paris: Masson)
7. Fishel, A. (1930). Uber die Entwicklung der Keimdrüsen des Menschen. *Z. Anat. Entwickl. (Kl). Gesch.*, **92**, 34
8. Pinkerton, J. A. M., McKay, D. G., Adams, E. C. and Hertig, A. T. (1961). Development of the human ovary. *Obstet. Gynecol.*, **18**, 152
9. Gruenwald, P. (1942). The development of the sex cords in the gonads of man and mammals. *Am. J. Anat.*, **70**, 359
10. Torrey, T. W. (1945). The development of urogenital system of the albino rat. The gonads. *Am. J. Anat.*, **76**, 375
11. Merchant, H. (1975). Rat gonadal and ovarian organogenesis with and without germ cells. *Dev. Biol.*, **44**, 1
12. Waldeyer, W. (1870). *Eierstock und EI*. (Liepzig: Engleman)
13. Witschi, E. (1962). *Embryology of the Ovary*. Academy of Pathology Monographs, Vol. 3, p. 1. (Baltimore: Williams and Wilkins)
14. Reeves, G. (1980). Stromal and follicular compartments of the ovary. Their influence in the development and involution of the organ. In Tozzini, R. I., Reeves, G. and Pineda, R. L (eds.) *Endocrine Physiopathology of the Ovary*, p. 137. (Amsterdam: Elsevier/North-Holland Biomedical Press)
15. Zamboni, L., Bezard, J. and Mauleon, P. (1980). The role of mesonephros in the development of the mammalian ovary. In Tozzini, R. I., Reeves, G. and Pineda, R. L. (eds.) *Endocrine Physiopathology of the Ovary*. (Amsterdam: Elsevier/North-Holland Biomedical Press)
16. Anderson, E. (1977). Junctional complexes in the developing ovarian follicle and the pre-implantation mammalian embryo with particular reference to gap junctions. *Res. Reprod.*, **9**, 5
17. Pedersen, T. (1972). Follicle growth in the mouse ovary. In Biggers and Schultz (eds.) *Oogenesis*, p. 361. (Baltimore: University Park Press)
18. Richards, J. S., Ireland, J. J., Rao, M. C., Bernath, G. A., Midgley, A. R. and Reichert, L. E. Jnr. (1976). Ovarian follicular development in the rat: hormone receptor regulation by estradiol, FSH and LH. *Endocrinology*, **99**, 1562
19. Richards, J. S. (1980). Maturation of ovarian follicles: actions and interactions of pituitary and ovarian hormones on follicular cell differentiation. *Physiol. Rev.*, **60**, 51
20. Gougeon, A. (1981). *Critique de la Croissance et de l'involution des Follicules Ovariens Pendant le Cycle Menstruel Chez la Femme*. Thèse de Doctorat d'Etat es Sciences Naturelles. Université de Paris VI
21. Dubreuilh, G. (1947). *La Glande Thécale de l'Ovaire Féminin. Conception d'Ensemble*. (Paris: C.R. Ass. des Anatomistes)
22. Dubreuilh, G. (1957). Le déterminisme de la glande thécale de l'ovaire. Induction morphogène à partir de la granulosa folliculaire. *Acta Anatomica*, **30**, 269
23. Feinberg, R. (1981). Thecosis. In Sommers, S. and Rosen P. P. (eds.) *Pathology Annual*, Part 2. (New York: Appleton-Century-Crofts)
24. McNatty, K. P., Makris, A., de Grazia, C., Osathanondh, R. and Ryan, K. J. (1979). The production of Pg, androgens, estrogens by granulosa cells, thecal tissue, and stroma tissue from human ovaries *in vitro*. *J. Clin. Endocrinol. Metab.*, **49**, 687
25. Byskov, A. G. (1978). In Jones, R. E. (ed.) *The Vertebrate Ovary. Comparative Biology and Evolution*, p. 533. (New York: Plenum Press)
26. Roddick, J. W. and Greene, R. R. (1957). Relation of ovarian stromal hyperplasia to endometrial carcinoma. *Am. J. Obstet. Gynecol.*, **73**, 843

8
The menopausal ovary

C. Gompel and N. Kitt

Several decades ago it was considered unusual to receive a histological specimen containing a post-menopausal ovary. It has been estimated that during the seventeenth century the chance of a woman reaching the age of menopause was 25% and by the nineteenth century it had only reached 50%. Today in the industralized countries approximately 95% of all women survive to the menopause.

What are the mechanisms that bring about the histological changes that are progressively observed in the ovary during the pre-menopausal period?

The large number of ovocytes that are present at birth slowly decreases, either by reaching maturation or by a process of degeneration during the sexual years. Not only does the number of ovocytes decrease, but their viability diminishes. This deterioration of both the quantity and the quality of the ovocytes leads to a diminution in the production of oestradiol, which is necessary for the maturation of the follicles.

This results in a shortening of the menstrual cycle which occurs at the expense of the follicular phase, as well as an increase in the FSH secretion in an attempt to stimulate a larger number of follicles. The secretion of LH remains normal at first and results in a luteal phase which is unchanged.

As the follicular atresia progresses, the level of FSH continues to increase, the oestrogen level decreases and the level of LH finally rises in response to the fall in steroid levels.

These high FSH levels are characteristic of the menopause. Because of the variability in the number of ovocytes remaining at the time of menopause, it is not possible to predict at what age it will occur.

The complex histology of the ovary explains the various modifications seen at the time of menopause. These changes occur progressively and at a rhythm that varies with each individual.

It has been noted that the follicular maturation ends and there is a decrease in the production of a corpus luteum. In a study by Bonfirraro involving 43 menstruating women between the ages of 45 and 53[1], it was shown that only two-thirds of them had a corpus luteum. In addition, when present, they were shown to be qualitatively deficient; the endometrium of these women did not demonstrate any luteal activity. And when there were signs of luteal activity, it could be attributed to luteinized stromal cells and not to a functional corpus luteum.

After the age of 50, it is possible to observe a few remaining ovocytes and follicles in the ovary of a menopausal woman. However, even if they have a normal histological appearance, they are probably non-viable. Some of these follicles degenerate into follicular cysts. These are usually few in number and are no larger than 0.5 cm in diameter.

A functional Graafian follicle persisting after menopause is rare. Numerous studies have confirmed the absence of ovulation after 52 years of age. A few cases of functional ovaries with persistent ovulation have been reported after the age of 50. Dawood et al.[2] reported finding a recent corpus luteum and normal follicles in a 65-year-old woman who underwent a hysterectomy for uterine fibromas. The endometrium in this case was of a secretory type. This woman had a history of chronic alcoholism as well as taking oral oestrogens, two factors which will lower FSH and LH levels.

The question of ovarian oestrogen production in the post-menopausal woman is somewhat beyond the object of this discussion. However, it must be noted in order to understand the histology of the menopausal ovary. In addition, the existence at all of ovarian oestrogen production is still a controversial subject.

The demonstration of a specific dehydrogenase and ultrastructural modifications of ovarian cells of the hilus and cortical stroma of menopausal woman would suggest that these cells are capable of steroid synthesis. Oestrogen production occurs either directly from these cells or by conversion from androgens. The peripheral conversion of oestrogens from androstenedione is therefore not the only source of oestrogens.

The ultrastructural modifications noted in these cells consist of the presence of mitochondria rich in cristae and of an abundance of smooth endoplasmic reticulum. These structures are also found in other cells which are active in the production of steroids, especially cells found in the granulosa.

It is difficult to appreciate by simple histological examination the ageing and structural alterations of ovocytes. They can, however, be demonstrated by the appearance of a series of genetic abnormalities that can be demonstrated by some examples such as: Down's syndrome, trisomy 21 or mongolism; Patau's syndrome or trisomy 13; Edward's syndrome or trisomy 18. These are all characterized by the addition of one chromosome or chromosome fragment on to the pair of chromosomes that define the syndrome.

The syndromes of Klinefelter and of Triplex, characterized by anomalies of the sex chromosomes, are also related to ovarian ageing. However, this does not seem to be the case for Turner syndrome.

The histological modifications which are observed during the menopause occur progressively. The ovarian cortex can atrophy or on the contrary can present diffuse or nodular hyperplasia. In the case of atrophy, the cells are small, the nuclei elongated and there is an increase in the amount of collagen fibres.

Hyperplasia or proliferation of the ovarian stroma begins as isolated islands deep in the cortical and medullary stroma. These islands grow progressively, joining to form voluminous nodules. One can readily identify these cells by the presence of a clear, slightly eosinophilic cytoplasm and an elongated enlarged nucleus with fuzzy borders. Some cells acquire an abundant cytoplasm which corresponds to the phenomenon of luteinization. Some cells show the presence of an increased enzymatic activity when examined histochemically. These cells frequently take the shape of spirals or ribbons.

This hyperplasia can be diffuse or form nodules large enough to distort the ovarian cortex. When they are discrete their presence is not easy to evaluate and includes an element of subjectivity. The coexistence of cortical hyperplasia with endometrial carcinoma, breast cancer, the presence of virilism or other conditions such as obesity or renal angiosclerosis has been found to be statistically significant. The aetiology of this hyperplasia is poorly understood. The data obtained on the endocrinological activity associated with this type of hyperplasia has suggested that it is androgenic in nature. The fact that peripheral transformation of androgens to oestrogens occurs explains why there is an association between cortical hyperplasia and hyperoestrogenic states.

The presence of isolated luteal cells or cells forming small islets in the cortical or the medullary stroma is noted before the menopause. The term thecomatosis is applied to these islets. When these cells are found disseminated throughout a hyperplastic stroma, it is called hyperthecosis. These cells are noted in a variety of endocrine and metabolic conditions such as obesity, hypertension, hirsutism, abnormal glucose metabolism and menstrual irregularities. They are more frequently noted in the ovaries of post-menopausal women who are otherwise normal. They are in fact found in 25% of post-menopausal ovaries.

These luteal islets are sometimes small. It is necessary to be somewhat lucky to locate them. Especially if only a limited number of slides are examined.

The aetiology of these luteal cells, as well as the cortical proliferation, is obscure. The activity of the gonadotrophic hormones could partially explain this anomaly.

The presence of cortical granulomas is observed in approximately 15% of ovaries examined. They consist of epitheloid cells, lymphocytes, multinucleated giant cells and occasionally lipid crystals. They can arise from abnormal coelomic inclusion cysts or from islets of endometrial stroma in the ovarian cortex.

Some studies have also demonstrated the presence of granular cells (K cells of Hamperl). This could tend to favour the endometrial origin of these granulomas.

Wallart has described fibrous bodies or zones of hyalinization in post-menopausal ovaries. These increase in frequency with age and are a common finding in women over 60 years of age. The tinctorial properties of these zones, which show a weakly positive staining with orcein, are consistent with the presence of elastic fibres. These zones probably represent scarring as a result of the previously described granulomatous lesions.

The hilar or Leydig's cells are observed in more than 80% of post-menopausal ovaries.

When carefully searched for by performing several sections at different levels of the organ, they tend to form small masses. They have round nuclei with finely granulated chromatin and a clear eosinophilic cytoplasm, in which occasionally a crystallized protein (crystalloid of Reinke) can be found. There appears to be a relationship between the abundance of these hilar cells and the intensity of the cortical hyperplasia. Likewise, there is a larger number of hilar cells in multiparous women, suggesting that there is a proliferation of these cells induced by the gonadotrophic hormones, the effect of which is noted after the menopause.

However, there seems to be no relationship between the number of hilar cells and any clinical manifestations related to androgens.

Rarely, ectopic islets of decidua have been observed in the ovaries of a post-menopausal woman. Usually, this can be explained by the presence of a trophoblastic tumour or by a woman treated with a progestational agent. In some cases, this occurrence cannot be explained and the endometrium of these women shows no evidence of progesterone effect. This variation could be explained by an increased sensitivity of the ovarian stroma to progestational stimulation.

Finally, the ovarian vessels will show evidence of ageing and arteriosclerosis, consistent with the generalized ageing process.

Before concluding this discussion, it should be noted that certain tumours become more frequent with advancing age. This is particularly true of the serous and mucinous carcinomas as well as metastases to the ovaries. Is the ageing of the ovary responsible for this increased frequency of ovarian tumours or is it secondary to the generalized ageing process? It is not possible to offer a definitive answer to this question, just as it is impossible to explain the exact reason for the cellular ageing process. If ageing can be considered as an alteration of the control of cellular differentiation, then the cessation of ovarian activity may be considered as a loss of the cellular function in the active structure of the organ.

References

1. Bonfirraro, G. and Subrizi, D. A. (1966). Aleune osservazioni sulla struttura dell' ovaia umana nella premenopausa. *Riv. Ostet. Ginecol.*, **21**, 433
2. Dawood, M. Y., Strongin, M., Krammer, E. E., *et al.* (1980). Recent ovulation in post menopausal woman. *Int. J. Gynaecol. Obstet.*, **18**, 192
3. Boss, J. H., Scully, R. E., Wegner, K. H. and Cohen, R. B. (1965). Structural variations in the adult ovary. Clinical significance. *Obstet. Gynecol.*, **25**, 747
4. Boyd, J. D. and Hamilton, W. J. (1955). The cellular components of the human ovary. In Bowes, K. (ed.) *Modern Trends in Obstetrics and Gynecology*. 2nd series. (London: Butterworth)
5. Chang, R. J. and Judd, H. L. (1981). The ovary after menopause. *Clin. Obstet. Gynecol.*, **24**, 181
6. Kemmann, E., Orenstein, D., Smith, C., *et al.* (1980). Estrogenization in women with postmenopausal ovarian hyperthecosis. *Int. J. Gynaecol. Obstet.*, **18**, 188
7. Krouse, T. B. (1980). In Eskin, B. A. (ed.) *Menopausal Pathology during The Menopause*. (New York: Masson)
8. Serment, H., Laffargue, P. and Vallette, C. (1969). *Press. Méd.*, **46**, 1653

9
The ovarian stroma after the menopause: activity and ageing

R. Loubet, A. Loubet and M-J. Leboutet

The post-menopausal (PM) period is marked by the disappearance of all cyclical activity in the hypothalamo-hypophyseal–ovarian axis, and by the gradual cessation of normal ovarian oestrogen secretion.

There is, however, no strict uniformity among the female population at the menopause: some women for a long time retain a hormone level which is low but sufficient to maintain some receptor trophicity[1]. Furthermore, PM development of androgen secretion is frequently evidenced by varying degrees of hirsutism.

Finally, in pathological cases, receptor anomalies may occur, resulting in ovarian functional hyperactivity (FH)

The origin of these PM hormone secretions was long a subject for discussion. Since it no longer had any follicular activity, the PM ovary seemed at first sight to have no further role to play and it was assumed that the hormone secretion was adrenal in origin. A long series of studies has shown that the ovary maintains its endocrine activity for a long time during the PM period[1-10].

Though questioned by some[11], experimental proof was first provided by castration, which results in a fall in the level of steroid hormones[1,4].

Precise results were later obtained by catheterizing the ovarian and peripheral veins and using radioimmunoassay (RIA) to measure the effects of stimulation and suppression[1,10,12,13] and by *in vitro* culture techniques.

MATERIAL

The present investigation is based on:

(1) 17 cases studied by light (LM) and electron microscopy (EM) in which morphological changes in uterine receptors show anachronistic oestrogen over-impregnation, attributable to functional hyperactivity of the PM ovarian stroma.

(2) One case of particular interest in a 75-year-old woman.

(3) The systematic study of a group of 30 PM ovaries (selected from subjects aged 50–84), whatever their external appearance or routine histology.

AIMS

Our aims were:

(1) To demonstrate the reality of steroid secretion over the entire PM period (4 years after the cessation of menses and for $\geqslant 20$ years).
(2) To establish a correlation between certain receptor changes and the morphological appearance of the ovarian stroma, with a definition of pathological states (hyperplasia and 'tumours').
(3) To try to specify the steroid function of the PM ovary and the nature of the hormones produced.
(4) To drawn attention to the role in gland ageing of deteriorating stromal blood vessels.

SIGNS OF STROMAL HYPERACTIVITY

In our series, PM stromal hyperactivity was identified in the uterus from the following signs:

(1) Diffuse endometrial hyperplasia.
(2) Areas of localized polypoid hyperplasia on involuting or atrophic mucous membrane, showing unequal endometrial receptivity. Despite its great oestrogen sensitivity (quantities of the order of 1 μg of 17β-oestradiol are enough to produce an oestrogen effect[5]), the endometrium ages and 'disconnects itself from the ovarian hormones'[7].
(3) Lesions of atypical hyperplasia.
(4) In 17 cases, an adenocarcinoma (ADK) of the endometrium found in association with hyperplasia or atrophy (during examination of the surgical specimen).

All these various repercussions in the uterine receptor were found together in a case of particular interest, a 75-year-old woman who had gone through the menopause at 50 and in whom curettage for metrorrhagia revealed glandular, polypoid, hyperoestrogenic and highly proliferative hyperplasia, and areas of atypical hyperplasia.

Examination at the time of the operation revealed a patient remarkable for a physical appearance much younger than her real age: her face was full and healthy, she had very few wrinkles, her breasts were firm, of average volume and with a pigmented areola.

The uterus was elastic and globular, weighing 140 g and measuring $120 \times 70 \times 40$ mm; the endometrium was 20 mm thick.

Histopathology showed, in addition to diffuse oestrogenic hyperplasia and areas of atypical hyperplasia, many large areas of florid uterine endometriosis, with a large number of active glands, and an abundant cytogenic chorion, loosely reticular in appearance and richly vascularized, dotted with haemorrhagic spots.

The ovaries were small (18×8 mm and 18×7 mm) and pinkish; their surface was smooth. Sections showed the tissue to be fleshy and light-brown to pinkish in colour, and succulent in appearance. It was homogeneous. There were no cysts, nor any nodular or tumour-like formations. On stained mid-ovary section, the whole gland appeared taken over by sarcomatoid stroma (0.8 cm).

All these findings testify to oestrogen hyper-stimulation, the level of which no doubt had happy consequences aesthetically speaking, but which nonetheless brought about an anachronistic uterine pathology together with, in the ovaries, an associated diffuse stromal hyperplasia, without any adenomatoid nodules or tumours.

It was this case which prompted us to undertake a systematic study of PM ovarian stroma activity, basing our work on the LM and EM study of ovaries from 30 selected subjects who had not undergone any hormone or radiation treatment (ages 50–80 years).

PM STROMAL ENDOCRINE ACTIVITY

The notion of PM ovarian endocrine function connected to stromal steroidogenic activity was first put forward in 1942 by Wallart[14], who pointed out that some ovaries retained a large volume of cortical tissue in the late PM period and that these cells were morphologically similar to those of the period of genital activity.

The stages in the increasing knowledge gained in this field were marked by several studies[5, 8–10, 15–23].

Proof of this steroidogenic activity is based on histomorphological arguments—ultrastructural (US) and cytoenzymological—on recent methods of biophysiological investigation with comparative hormone concentrations measured by RIA, and on the setting up of stromal cultures with or without gonadotrophic stimulation.

MACROSCOPIC FINDINGS

PM ovaries can be classified into three groups, according to their type:

Type 1—Smooth ovaries, of a volume that may be: normal; rather low, but with the normal shape retained; or conversely, in a state of harmonious hypertrophy. On section, the cortex is thick and shows up dark on stained whole-organ midline section, with frequent excursions towards the hilus.

Type 2—Retracted, somewhat wrinkled ovaries that are smaller than normal; 'fibro-atrophic' in appearance; pitted and deeply furrowed, showing a thin cortical layer on whole-organ midline section.

Type 3—Small, wrinkled, hard, flat, ivory-white or pearl-coloured ovaries; with deep incisions dividing the gland into irregular lobules; a very thin or even invisible stromal layer; a weight always much less than 10 g[24].

If type 1 generally corresponds to proven stromal hyperplasia, the common types 2 and 3 do not allow any presumptions to be made about the level of stromal functional activity.

More than the weight and general measurements of the gland[25, 26], it is the precise measurement in millimetres of cortical thickness on whole-organ midline haematoxylin- and eosin-stained section that in our opinion provides the most reliable criterion:

(1) Average readings for the 'normal' PM ovary vary from 0.3 to 1 mm.

(2) If $\geqslant 2$ mm thick, the signs of functional hyperplasia (FH) must be sought with the help of supplementary staining (lipid staining).
(3) If $\geqslant 2.5$ mm thick, FH must be considered established (for comparison, the average cortical thickness of a normal young ovary is 8–10 mm).

Note that the ovary always thins to the detriment of the medullary stroma, which accounts for the surface wrinkling of the gland.

HISTOMORPHOLOGY UNDER CONVENTIONAL LM

In the normal PM period, the narrow fibrous layer on the surface (wrongly referred to as the 'albuginous' layer) loses its individuality.

Beneath, the medullary stromal/hilar boundary moves closer to the surface: it is often jagged or irregular, owing to deep conical or nodular expansions of the stroma; this brings about some fusion between the two areas.

For the 20 years of the PM period, the thinner stroma, which has moved closer to the surface, retains a 'sarcomatoid stroma' appearance, i.e. it is fairly cellular tissue that still contains, for 2–4 years after menstruation has ceased, a few primordial follicles[27,28] that can still be stimulated (Lunenfeld).

PM STROMAL CYTOMORPHOLOGY

Under LM at a magnification of 900, three types of cells can be distinguished in this fibroblastic stroma[26]:

(1) Narrow, stretched and elongated fibroblastic-type cells, with a long, thin nucleus densely packed with cromatin.
(2) Equally slender cells, but more dumpy, with a broader, abundant cytoplasm which is light and sometimes vacuolated, with a larger, oval and nucleolated nucleus, containing dispersed chromatin. These cells can easily be located by staining with Sudan IV: this shows up their lipid content and locates them in a 'stromal lipid band'[17] which is in fact fairly broken. This 'band' tends to move down towards the hilum as the cortex gets thinner.
(3) Globular epithelioid cells, 20–35 μm in diameter, with a broad pale cytoplasm bounded by a distinct membrane. The nucleus is large, spherical and central, with fine chromatin and a large nucleolus. Staining with black Sudan IV or osmic acid makes them easily visible: Schultz colouring gives uneven results[26]. These large thecostromal cells are: (i) not always found; (ii) isolated; (iii) found together in small groups of 3–6, when they are easily recognized by their light cytoplasm which earned them the name they were given by Scully[29]: 'stromal luteinized cells'. They may be compared with smaller, equally epithelioid cells which readily group together in lines that are often perpendicular to the gland surface. The cytoplasm of these cells is eosinophilic, their nucleus is smaller and their chromatin denser. These small thecal-epithelioid-type cells may also be found in association with FH.

Between these various cell types, intermediates may be found:

(1) The environment is made up of blood vessels and collagen; the latter tends to become more plentiful with age.

(2) Macro-microscopic correlation is good for the macro type 1, especially for glands with a cortex of 2 mm; it is particularly in these glands that the small groups of 'luteinized stromal or thecal cells' are found, giving a 'post-menopausal thecomatosis-like' appearance (Fraenkel[3] created the term 'hyperthecosis'). A morphological variation is *nodular stromal hyperplasia*, which can give a pseudo-tumorous appearance: the gland is enlarged and deformed, with a lumpy surface[16, 30].

Finally, in this group come the majority of cases of diffuse stromal hyperplasia (SH): ovaries of normal size and shape with a uniformly thick spindle cell stroma and abundant lipid content shown on staining. Collagen content is low, and there are surfaces or nodules of stromal extension in the medullohilar region.

Types 2 and 3 do not correlate well: in the majority of cases they correspond to PM glands with an average functional level, but cases of FH can be found among them (usually in patients suffering from late metrorrhagia—endometrial oestrogenic hyperplasia—hirsutism).

It is in type 3 glands that histochemical lipid location is the most necessary; cortical retraction and dense collagen may mask real functional activity.

ULTRASTRUCTURE OF PM OVARIAN STROMA

Ultrastructural studies confirm the existence of:

—a dual cell population, made up of fibroblastic and steroidogenic cells, and
—the passage from one type to the other via a group of intermediary cells.

Semi-fine localizing sections proved an excellent method for rapidly identifying:

—slender, fibroblastoid lipid-storing cells, as well as those with a low lipid content;
—Scully's 'luteinized' epithelioid cells, which are often scarce and scattered over a large area.

Quantitative assessment of optically significant cells is made possible by this method, even in the most 'fibrous' ovaries.

US CHARACTERISTICS OF FUNCTIONAL STROMAL CELLS

Functional stromal cells are easily told apart from fibroblasts by their morphology and organelles; and by their environment.

US morphology

(a) Slender but polymorphous cells
These are:

Long (12–15 µm). The cytoplasm has many extensions, which intermingle with those of neighbouring cells.

There is simple cell contact, without desmosomes; however, fibroblastic tonofilaments have been observed in some instances[20].

Pinocytosis has been described in the membrane; in our material, this was found particularly in a few rare myofibroblasts. These may be found in conjunction with the muscle cells observed under LM by Wallart[14], and with the 'contractile cells' found in the stroma by Ross and Schreiber (reference 31, p. 65).

The long nucleus is often irregular and indented, which accounts for the frequency of cytoplasmic pseudo-inclusions. Heterochromatin is dispersed, and may be found concentrated in linear fashion along the nuclear membrane.

The nucleolus is bulky, and filamentous in appearance.

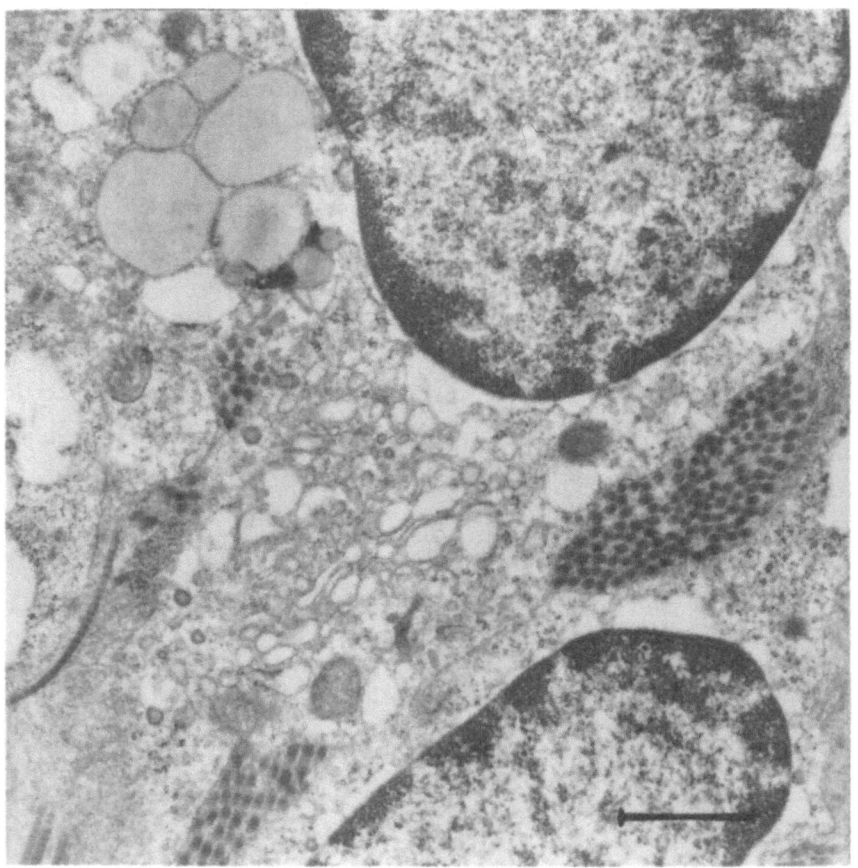

Figure 1   Post-menopausal stromal hyperplasia in a 75-year-old woman. Cell with Golgi apparatus, abundant smooth reticulum, ribosomes and low density lipids.   ——— = 1 µm

Cell elements—These are abundant and are found grouped together to form a variety of functional compounds (Figure 1):

Free ribosomes or polyribosomes.

Highly developed Golgi bodies, with many microvesicles.

Abundant, twisted and frequently dilated endoplasmic reticulum (ER), particularly smooth ER.

Mitochondria are either normal in size and morphology, or else bulky (0.5–0.8 µm), in which case they possess a dense matrix and tubular crests which are quite characteristic. No inclusions were found here.

Lipid inclusions—Lipid inclusions are always to be found in functional cells, where they make up the most characteristic element. But in their number, electron density and morphology they vary greatly, and this may be related to the functional importance of the cell. The two-fold classification proposed by P. Laffargue *et al.*[20] is still valid:

Type I—Average or low density inclusions. Droplets with an average diameter of 0.8 µm and a three-leaved membrane which is sometimes quite distinct and other times invisible, in which case it gives the appearance of a diffuse stain.

Type II—Dense, heterogeneous inclusions containing very dense grains of lipofuscin, various granular inclusions, and myelinoid bodies.

Inclusions of type I readily form functional compounds with mitochondria, dilated smooth ER tubules, and the nucleus. Functional couplings are identical with those described in other steroid cells (theca, Leydig, adrenal)[32]. This lipid material forms the raw material for steroid biosynthesis[33]. Type II inclusions accompany degeneration: accumulation of the by-products of steroid synthesis, in the case of hyperfunctional cells[34], and the products of unsaturated fatty acid auto-oxidation, in the case of cells with an average, late PM-type, functional level[20, 35].

(b) Thecostromal epithelioid cells

So-called 'luteinized cells' were found in ovaries with FH, even late in the PM period (six cases).

Identified as theca cells in 1965 in rats by Sato[36], they were studied in women by Hertig[15]. In our material they appeared with an abundance of polyribosomes, a large number of tubular crested mitochondria and an abundant, dilated smooth ER, explaining the light appearance of the cytoplasm. Lipid inclusions were rare, small and homogeneously pale, as in type I (Figure 2).

In our series of PM ovaries unassociated with FH, we found somewhat different appearances:

(1) Dense-matrix, tubular-crested mitochondria were rare (but hardly ever totally absent).
(2) Poorer Golgi development.
(3) Predominance of dense and heterogeneous lipid inclusions (type II), which were frequently abundant and bulky, so that they looked like storage cells; compounds of lipid, mitochondria, nucleus and smooth ER were rare; lipofuscin was abundant.

We may add that a stromal cell containing a crystalloid was described in a case of FH by Adechi-Benkoel[37]; and microperoxysomes were described by Familiari *et al.*[38].

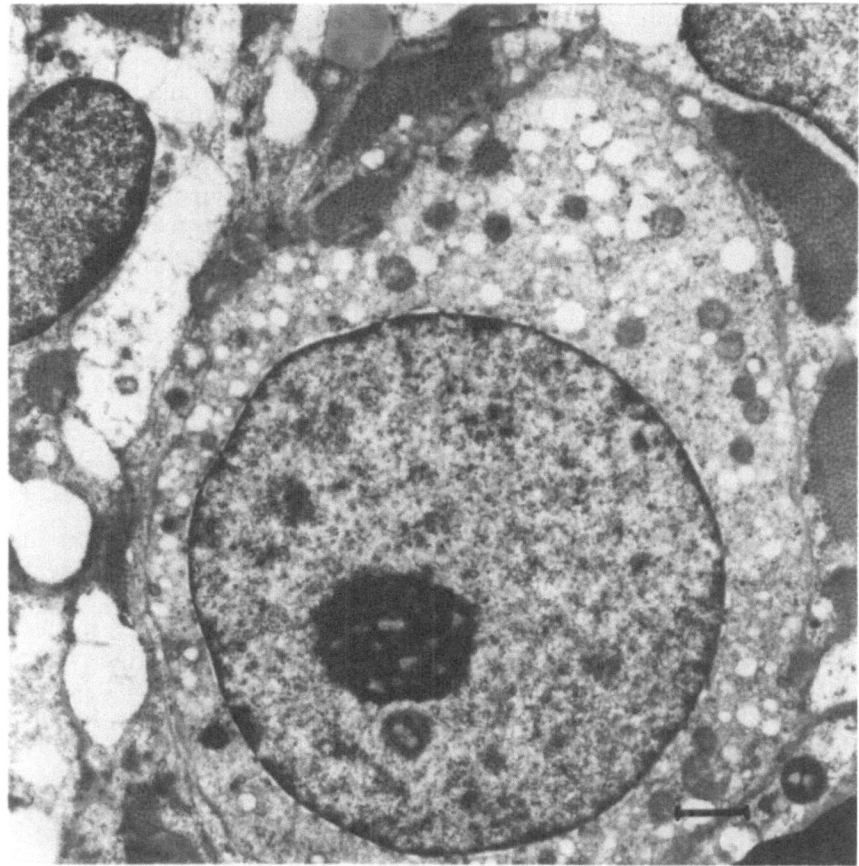

Figure 2 Thecostromal epithelioid cell. Round or oval cell. Large round nucleus with large nucleolus. Abundant and dilated smooth reticulum. Mitochondria. ———— = 1 μm

(c) Fibroblasts

Supporting this population of functional or potentially steroidogenic cells are a large number of fibroblasts; the number increases in late PM period ovaries, along with the rate of production of the collagen that makes up their immediate environment.

Their differential diagnosis is based on the length of the fibroblast, the density of its cytoplasm, the abundance of rough ER (RER) and the presence of intra-cytoplasmic filaments.

(d) Transition cells

Transition cells are frequent, though their morphology gives no clear indication of how they have evolved; features of both cell types may be found to coexist within them—fibroblasts (collagen production, areas of intracytoplasmic collagen) and steroid cells (polyribosomes, a large number of lamellar-crested mitochondria, well-developed Golgi, lipid vesicles and many lipid-mitochondria compounds). Lipofuscin content seemed related to dedifferentiation (as in our type 3 hilar cell (HC)[39]).

(e) Cells in cytolysis

Some cells were observed undergoing cytolysis. These cells were packed with autophagic structures (lysosomes, residual bodies, GR membrane fragments). Mitochondria were swollen and their crests effaced. ER was stretched and vacuolated. There was homogenization and densification of chromatin.

These degenerational features seemed commoner in ovaries with a high functional level.

The large quantity of lipid released in cytolysis prompts us to point out its role in the development of cortical granuloma, as described under LM by Woll, Hertig and Johnson[30], and which are common in this type of gland.

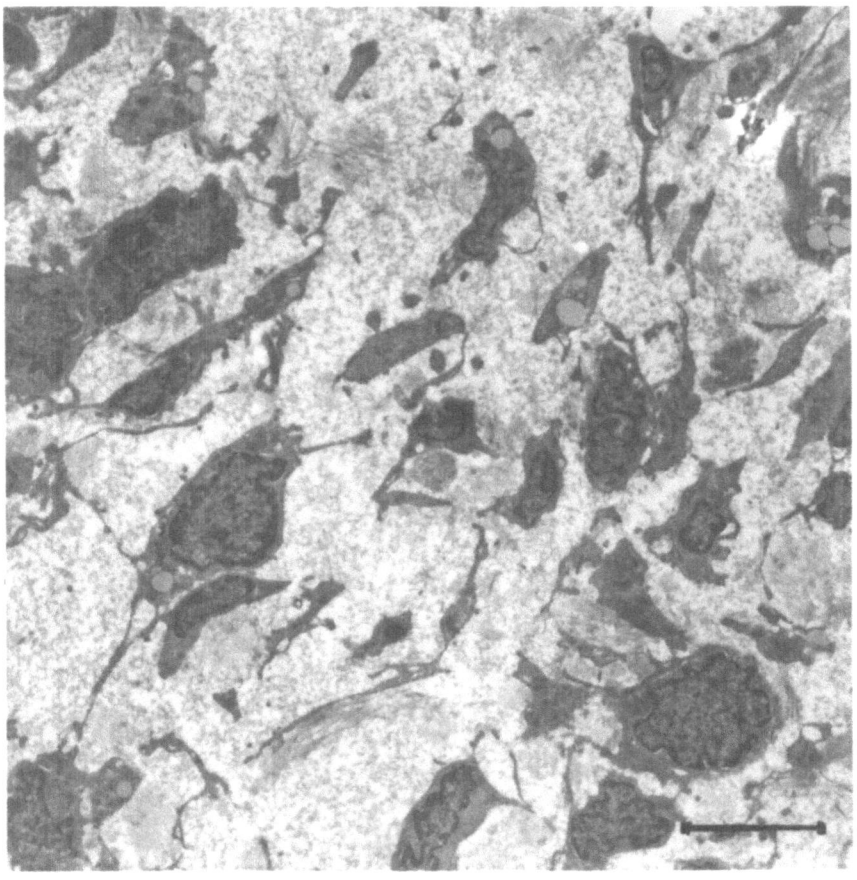

Figure 3 Post-menopausal stroma. Cells scattered in plentiful collagen. Intracellular lipids (storage cells). ———— = 5 μm

Thus there is a range of functional stromal cells identifiable at the ultrastructural level, mixed in with the fibroblasts, with a reversible relationship existing between two fundamental types:

(1) Cells in full metabolic activity which are low in lipid inclusions and high in specific cell elements, corresponding to Balboni's SPC ('steroid producing cell')[40].

(2) Quiescent (storage) cells with a concentration of cholesterol, triglycerides, phospholipids and cholesterol esters[18], commoner in late PM ovaries with no signs of FH; they correspond to cells with an incomplete enzyme complement.

The cell environment—The abundance of collagen is inversely proportional to stromal functional activity (Figures 3 and 4). The relationship between functional cells and blood vessels proved of particular interest. In active stromal glands,

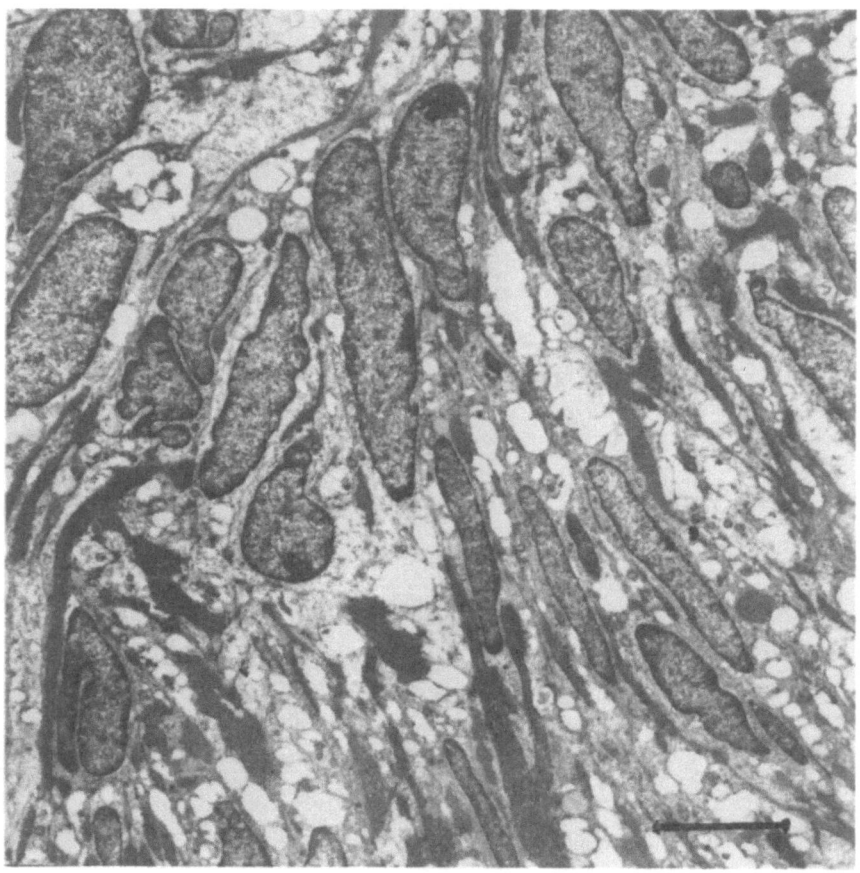

Figure 4 Stromal hyperplasia in a 75-year-old woman. Hypercellularity with low collagen. Low density lipids, frequently extracted. ——— = 5 μm

stromal cells undergoing steroidogenic differentiation tend to arrange themselves around a capillary, sometimes forming bands that are separated by an endocrine-type capillary network. Study of the immediate relationship between functional cell and blood vessel reveals a loose perivascular zone—a basal membrane which may be thick, and possibly layered around a capillary with glycogen and rich cytoplasm, but which is more commonly thin with, in FH ovaries, an extremely close link between the functional cell and the active endothelial cell: the vessel wall is of the sinusoid type, without pericytes. In such cases the endometrial cells are bulky and prominent: their nucleus is large and nucleolated, and there is intense pinocytosis forming a tight vesicular edge. Unlike P. Laffargue, we did not find any lipid inclusions migrating into the perivascular space; though sometimes a lipid vesicle was noted in the cytoplasm of a functional endothelial cell.

US morphology thus proves the existence of a stromal cell population showing signs of steroidogenic activity.

Histoenzymological methods may be used to specify the functional activity of these cells and the metabolic pathway they follow.

HISTOENZYMOLOGICAL DATA

Two methodologies comprise this technique[5,17–19,21,28,41,42].
—detection of intracellular enzyme systems;
—studies of the *in vitro* synthetic activity of stromal fragments, using various substrates, with or without gonadotrophic stimulation.

Detection of intracellular enzyme systems

Non-specific dehydrogenases—characteristic of the intermediary metabolism of cells engaged in intense synthetic activity are: G-6 PDH (pentose pathway), LDH (anaerobic glycolysis), NADH and NADPH diaphorases (respiratory chain).

Specific dehydrogenases of 'steroid label' steroid metabolism[21] are 3β-hydroxysteroid dehydrogenase (3βOHSD) and 17β-hydroxysteroid dehydrogenase. Their presence indicates the steroid maturity of the stroma cell. Once detected, a specific idea of the pathway followed in hormone synthesis can be gained by referring to the established steroidogenetic pathways:

(1) Δ_4-sterone pathway: via progesterone (P), catalysed by 17βOHSD, leading to Δ_4 androstenedione (A) then to testosterone (T) or oestrone (E_1) and in some cases 17β-oestradiol (E_2).

(2) Δ_5-sterol pathway: via DHA in the absence of 3βOHSD, leading to (A) then to the events shown in Figure 5.

(3) In a series of 14 PM ovaries (from subjects aged 52–81 years), P. Laffargue found that 78% of the glands contained enzymatically active cells (corresponding to Scully's EASC 'enzymatically active stromal cell'). The proportion is only 50% for young ovaries (stromal zones at some distance from follicular structures) with a limited quantity of EASC.

(4) During the menopausal transition period, 56% of the ovaries were found to be enzymatically active, with nests of thecoepithelioid cells in the superficial cortex and EASC in the deep stroma.

(5) In the late PM period, the EASC form into groups near the blood vessels deep in the cortex by the end of the hilum; they become impossible to tell apart from groups of HC, which themselves are often hyperplastic[39].

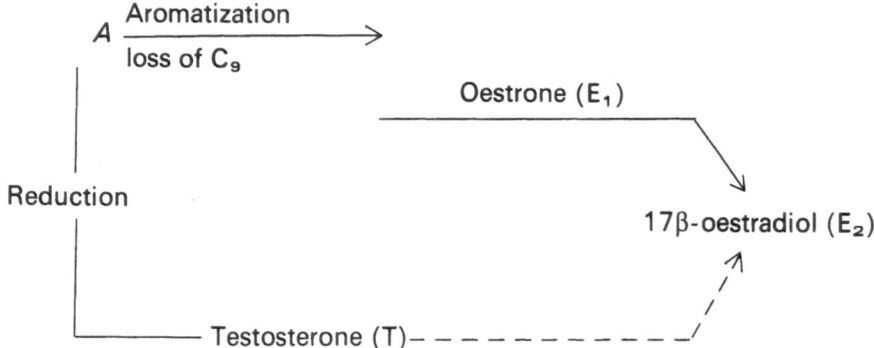

Figure 5 Formation of 17β-oestradiol from Δ_4 androstenedione in the sterol pathway

Morphologically functional cells with a high lipid content have, as a rule, an incomplete complement of enzyme systems (intermediary or storage cells).

However, a strict parallel cannot be drawn between morphological differentiation and the state of completeness of the enzyme systems. Enzyme action precedes morphological differentiation, and from this stems the whole interest of cyto-enzymology.

In vitro incubation

In vitro incubation of slices of stroma and substrate[5, 43] is undergoing investigation which is needed for an up-to-date understanding of the functional role of PM stroma.

STROMAL CELL HORMONOSYNTHESIS IN THE PM OVARY: ASSOCIATED PATHOLOGY

It has long been recognized that, with their steroidogenic morphology and histoenzymatic activity, stromal cells secrete oestrogen.

As early as 1938, Corner[44] had expertly shown how, in animals, the ovary continued to secrete oestrogen after irradiation had destroyed all the follicles but left the stroma intact.

Further evidence was forthcoming from receptor studies:

(1) In many women, receptor levels are retained to some degree over the PM period.
(2) Stromal functional hyperplasia occurs in association with endometrial hyperplasia, and this syndrome is a possible stage in the development of endometrial ADK.
(3) Urinary hormone assays, when carried out in the PM patient, show high oestrogen levels that fall after hysterectomy and castration[4].

This stromal oestrogen secretion which develops at the time when the folliculothecal source is drying up thus appears to take on the role of a substitute gland, maintained and prolonged by the continuous high levels of LH.

Further arguments were provided by the injection of hCH in PM women ('natural stimulation' of the stroma carried out in PM patients with endometrial ADK, aged 53–73, by Polyak *et al.*[45]), which gives the following results:

(1) A rise in urinary phenolsteroids and vaginal acidophilic levels.
(2) The appearance of large epithelioid cell nodules in the stroma.
(3) Nodular thecomatosis, of the type described by Fraenkel[3], and which was the subject of US and HZM studies by P. and F. Laffargue in 1969 and 1974.

Thus it was known that at too high a level, and especially if kept up for too long, natural PM gonadotrophic stimulation may induce diffuse or nodular stromal hyperplasia, sometimes of a pseudo-tumour-like nature: e.g. thecoma[46]. Our own series includes two small thecomas associated with diffuse contralateral SH, in two patients of 60 and 67 suffering from invasive endometrial ADK. The general shape of the ovaries had been preserved. The large and nodular lesion showed the intersecting fibrous bands that are characteristic of the cell mass; the frequency of such phenomena is perhaps underestimated from the US point of view. According to F. Laffargue, the cellular proliferation 'sums up, in a disordered and dystrophic fashion, the evolution of fibroblasts into steroid-secreting cells'.

For such a lesion to develop, it probably needs to be preceded by a stage of SH[46].

HZM studies on these thecomas since Pfleiderer and Teufel in 1968[49] have shown, paradoxically, that there is little 3βOHSD and that cell enzyme activity is low. Certainly, as far as the bulkier thecomas are concerned, it may be considered that the sheer mass of the cells makes up for the low activity of individual cells[47], or else that hormone synthesis is incomplete, or that it follows different pathways than in the normal ovary, e.g. the sulphate pathway suggested by Burstein and Dorfmann[48], which does not pass via 5-pregnenolone, but leads directly to oestrone instead, then to oestradiol, without any role being played by 3βOHSD.

Recent biophysiological techniques may be used to support hypotheses concerning the development of these thecomas. Such techniques include essentially:

(1) *In vitro* incubation of stromal tissue slices with radioactive substrates, with or without hCH stimulation.
(2) Cultures of various types of isolated cells[43].
(3) Ovarian and peripheral vein catheterization, comparing steroid levels in the venous effluent.
(4) *In vitro* and *in vivo* studies showing the role of peripheral tissues as major sites of steroid conversion[50, 51].

In 1966, Rice and Savard[5] showed, using *in vitro* incubation of stromal tissue slices, that normal ovarian stroma produces mainly androgens (androsterone, DHA testosterone) from [^{14}C]acetate. On a much smaller scale, and at a lower level, it produces oestrone and 17β-oestradiol.

This observation was confirmed in 1969 by Mattingly and Huang[52] and then by many others[1, 6, 8, 23, 53]. McNatty[23] concluded that normal or PM ovarian stroma produces mainly androstenedione, little oestradiol, only traces of oestrone, testosterone and dihydrotestosterone, and that surgical removal of the stroma reduces androgen secretion in cases of ovarian hyperandrogenism.

For Vermeulen[8] the PM ovary secretes neither oestrone nor oestradiol, the levels of these hormones remaining uninfluenced by ovariectomy or hCH stimulation; these results confirm those of Rader[54] and later of Judd[1] obtained by comparative catheterization of the ovarian and peripheral veins and in some cases by ovariectomy.

The predominance of androstenedione secretion accounts for the frequent development of PM hirsutism. In this context a comparison may be made between the stimulated PM ovary and the stromal hyperplasia found in the polycystic ovary syndrome, in which it has been known since the studies by Mahesh[55], Rivarola[51], Givens[56] and Geller[48] that the inappropriate LH or Interstitial Cell Stimulating Hormone (ICSH) secretion responsible for stromal hyperplasia leads to a significantly higher concentration of androgens in ovarian and peripheral blood than in normal women.

The absence of an hCG response in castrated women, the decline in LH activity and the rate of testosterone secretion in women on combined oestrogen–progestagen therapy all confirm the very important role played by the ovary in the pathogenesis of hirsutism[57, 58].

A study by Judd et al.[1] of testosterone, androstenedione, 17β-oestradiol and oestrone levels in blood samples obtained by catheterization of ovarian and peripheral veins showed that in the PM period ovarian vein concentrations compared with those in the peripheral circulation were 15 times higher for testosterone, four times higher for androstenedione, and two times higher for 17β-oestradiol and oestrone. Similar results were found by Botella–Llusia[42].

In this respect we should emphasize a frequent finding in our own material: the parallel hyperplasia of functional stromal cells and hilar cells (HC), which are known to secrete androgens[59]. Both hyperplasias have the same cause—pituitary LH-ICSH stimulation, which remains constant after the fall in oestrogen levels during the menopausal transition period. This stimulation can result in adenomatous hyperplasia of the HC, as can be frequently observed during this period[39].

In two of our 17 cases (subjects aged 60 and 71), a functional cell type II HC adenoma was found in association with active stromal hyperplasia, hyperoestrogenic-like uterine receptor stimulation and hirsutism.

LH INDUCTION OF GONADAL STRUCTURES

Similarly, gonadotrophin stimulation of the PM ovary can in some cases bring about the appearance of gonad-like structures which, in the opinion of some authors, are the starting point for endocrine tumours that appear later. Data in support of this idea were reported in 1969 by P. Laffargue[60] under the title 'Dysplasia responses of ovarian endocrine tumours'.

The most frequently found features (apart from cortical groups of granular cells, with Call–Exner bodies which we did not find) were:

(1) Bands of theca-like acidophil cells with tubular cavitations resembling tubes of arrhenoblastoma[61].

(2) HC pseudo-tumour-like adenomatous nodular hyperplasia associated with thecostromal cells in an adenomatous hilar–thecal compound (two of our cases) that is truly ambiguous when the two cell types cannot be told apart on grounds of morphology alone.

These appearances prove that the ovarian stroma retains its fundamental plasticity in the PM period and that it is a true mesonephrotic blastoma able, even during the PM period, to give rise to 'young' structures under the effect of LH stimulation.

THE ASSOCIATION BETWEEN FUNCTIONAL PM STROMAL HYPERPLASIA AND NON-ENDOCRINE OVARIAN TUMOURS

To designate this association, Morris and Scully[62] coined the somewhat elliptical expression 'ovarian tumour with functional stroma'.

In 1962, Si Chun Ming[63] compiled 70 cases of Brenner's tumour associated with hormone activity. Woodruff and Acosta[64] pointed out the existence of metrorrhagia in half out of 50 reported cases of Brenner's tumour.

Fox[65] found evidence of an oestrogen-stimulated endometrium in 25% of common serous and mucinous epithelial tumours.

Eddie[66] and Edwards et al.[67] pointed out a significant increase in urinary oestriol in common PM ovarian tumours.

Edman and McDonald[68] emphasized the association between the daily production of androstenedione 11.7 mg and oestrone 170 mu (by extra-ovarian aromatization) and mucinous cystadenoma, adenomatous endometrial hyperplasia and thecostromal hyperplasia.

Hamwi et al.[69] demonstrated the in vitro production of testosterone from progesterone by a virilizing Brenner's tumour, under the influence of hCG added to the medium.

F. Laffargue and later workers using EM and HZM found that the percentage of PM ovarian tumours showing stromal hormone activity was between 34 and 38%[47, 70–72]. Dermoid cysts are rarely mentioned in these studies[73].

In our own material, the conditions most commonly associated with dual cell and stromal HC hyperplasia are mucinous cysts and Brenner's tumours. The commonest US feature found in association with mature teratoma was HC hyperplasia.

To explain this stromal activity, whether or not it occurs in association with HC activity, different hypotheses have been put forward:

(1) Non-specific tumour stimulation of the ovarian stroma, as during the process of follicle maturation[74].
(2) The hypothetical action of local endocrine factors through 'inversion of cell polarity' in certain neoplasms[75].

Our own impression is that a predominant role is played by gonadotrophin stimulation, since the contralateral ovary often shows an associated degree of hilar-stromal hyperplasia.

ASSOCIATED EXTRA-OVARIAN MALIGNANT TUMOUR PATHOLOGY

This category of pathology is dominated by the association between functional stromal hyperplasia and endometrial ADK. For Fienberg[26], 87% of PM endometrial ADK come into this category.

ADK may develop in two basic ways: (1) on a background of diffuse or polypous endometrial hyperplasia with a transitional appearance that leaves no doubt as to the relationship; (2) in a receptive and stimulated area, with the rest of the endometrium being in a state of atrophy which, moreover, may have come about after the development of the ADK.

We should like to emphasize in passing the infiltrative character of our ADK which we have distinguished from cases of reversible atypical hyperplasia that may occur in a context of luteal insufficiency[76, 77].

The ovarian stroma may show:

(1) Approximately symmetrical diffuse bilateral hyperplasia.
(2) Groups, bands or heaps of thecomatosis[26] associated with an increase in the overall volume of stromal tissue (0.2 cm thick), using the criteria laid down by Bigelow[16].

—We have noted the frequency of associated HC hyperplasia.
—We must also recall an associated infiltrating endometrial ADK (in the case of our two small thecomas).

FUNCTIONAL STROMA AND BREAST CARCINOMA

We would draw attention only to the association between breast carcinoma and SH noted by Sommerhausen and Gompel[78].

THE NATURE OF PM STROMAL ENDOCRINE SECRETION

Two broad categories may be distinguished: (1) physiological PM ovarian steroid secretion; (2) pathological steroidogenesis, in such conditions as diffuse or adenomatous SH and induced thecoma.

The apparent contradiction stems from the fact that, in most cases of SH, receptor status results in oestrogen over-impregnation, whereas recent studies have shown that PM stromal steroidogenesis gives rise essentially to androgens.

As we have already seen, a number of hypotheses have resulted from the study of thecomas, which are usually oestrogenic in their actions. In 1970, Netter et al.[7] suggested that oestrogens could be produced from ovarian androgens by extra-ovarian aromatization.

The aromatizing capability of PM stroma itself appears very limited; it seems to produce only a small quantity of E_1 oestrone from androstenedione (A)[10, 80].

However, in PM stromal hyperplasia (PMSH) Dennefors et al.[10] found that the stroma produced significantly higher levels of oestrogens than normal stroma.

For many authors and recently for Botella-Llusia (1980)[42], the hyperoestrogenic effect of hyperplasic stroma or its functional tumours is attributable to the rapid peripheral conversion of the testosterone (T) produced by the cells.

The importance of this peripheral conversion of the androgens produced and secreted by the stromal cells (the most important of them being androstenedione in the PM ovary) has been a constant feature of studies published since the work of Tait[50], Lipsett[80], Rivarola[51] and Baird[12].

Longcope's work[6] (in vitro with human tissue, in vivo with animals) has shown the pre-eminent role of muscle and adipose tissue in metabolism and as sites for the conversion and inter-conversion of sex steroids. Together these two tissues appear responsible for 40–50% of androgen aromatization into oestrogens, with activity being slightly higher in muscle.

In the PM woman, the rate of conversion increases significantly with age:

(1) The increase in adipose tissue mass with age[81] might account for the increase in conversion[22,82] thus explaining the role of obesity as a predisposing factor in endometrial ADK.

(2) Nevertheless, the fairly rapid increase in PM peripheral aromatization seems to suggest that a major role is played by the rise in LH and its stabilization at a relatively high level[6]; indeed, Cedar[83] showed that in isolated placental tissue aromatization may be increased by LH perfusion.

(3) It is equally possible that at the intracellular level a role may be played by alterations in pH with age and in the DPM/DPNH ratio[6].

The ability of some ovaries to develop SH or an induced secretory tumour seems conditioned by the persistence of gonadotrophin receptivity: this is shown by the significant increase in cAMP after hCG stimulation of the stroma in FH[10].

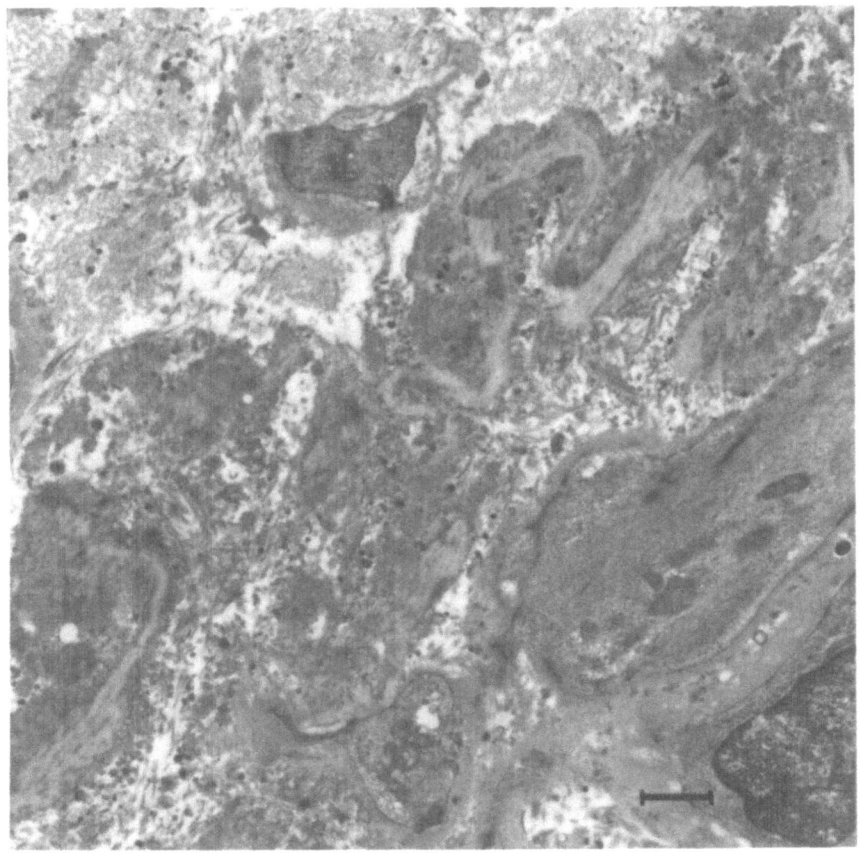

Figure 6 Elastolysis in intra-parenchymatous arteries. Elastic lamina keeps its general shape, but with thinning and gaps. ——— = 1 μm

cAMP acts as a mediator of gonadotrophic effect, though its exact mechanism of action in steroid synthesis has not yet been fully elucidated[84].

OVARIAN AND STROMAL INVOLUTION

In the involution of the ovary in general and more particularly of the ovarian stroma, one factor seems of prime importance: the small calibre arteries of the intra-parenchymatous functional sector (spiral arteries) are affected early on and begin to involute in much the same way as the vascular factor plays an essential role in the evolution of the corpus luteum (vascular penetration of the granulosa[85]).

These parenchymatous vessels are subject throughout life to the following:

Haemodynamic factors—Bringing into play the plasticity of this vascular network during cyclical events (luteogenesis), or episodic ones (pregnancy), resulting in enormous changes in profile, calibre and flow.

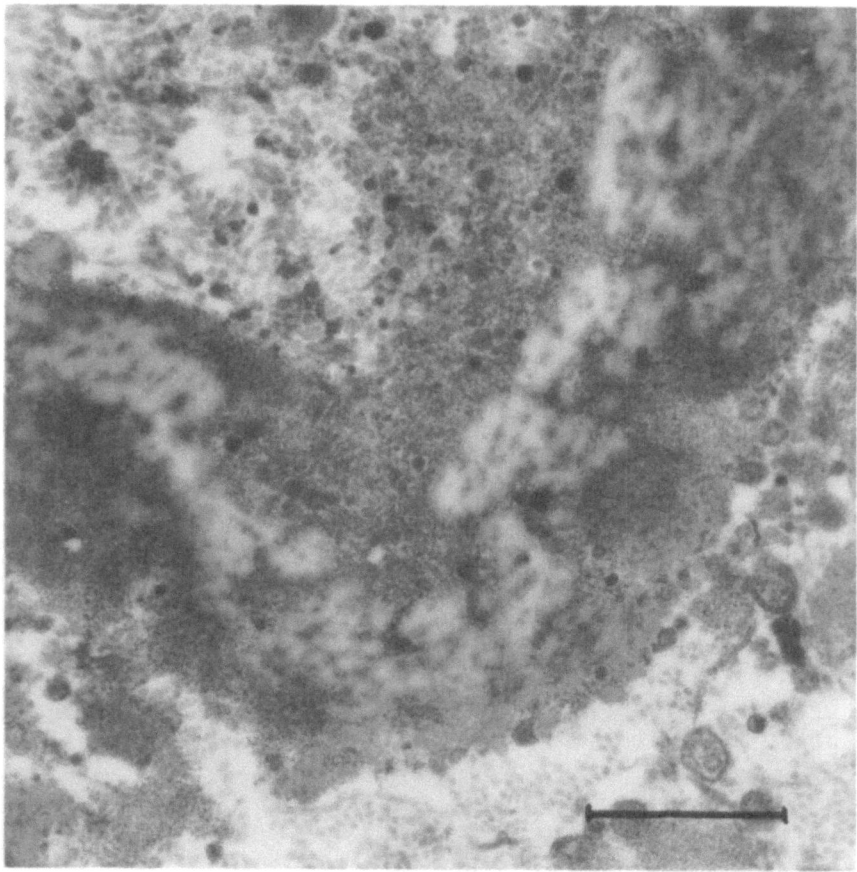

Figure 7 Elastolysis. Cloudy appearance and lacunar degeneration of elastin, which spreads in granulous substance. ——— = 1 μm

Endocrine factors—Such as the action of oestrogens on the development of the vascular network, its spiralization and its rapid adaptation to changes in circulatory conditions; the action of progesterone, which maintains blood flow at a sufficient level during the luteal phase and makes the blood vessels more sensitive to biogenic amines, as well as raising basal arterial tone (Kuhl); the action of the gonadotrophins, in expanding the capillary network and, secondarily, bringing about an increase in the calibre of the arteries[86, 87]; the prostaglandins (mainly PGF_2) which possibly lower progesterone levels without modifying total ovarian blood flow[88] (their luteolytic role has been experimentally confirmed by Baird[89] who found it to be associated with cybernins).

Unlike hilar arteries (the vascular supply sector) which show banal ageing lesions with advancing age, the helicoidal arteries of the intra-parenchymatous functional sector show a specific sequence of lesions[89]:

(1) Very early deterioration of the internal elastic lamina (stretching, folding into tight pleats, eroded contours); ultrastructural studies using Brissie's

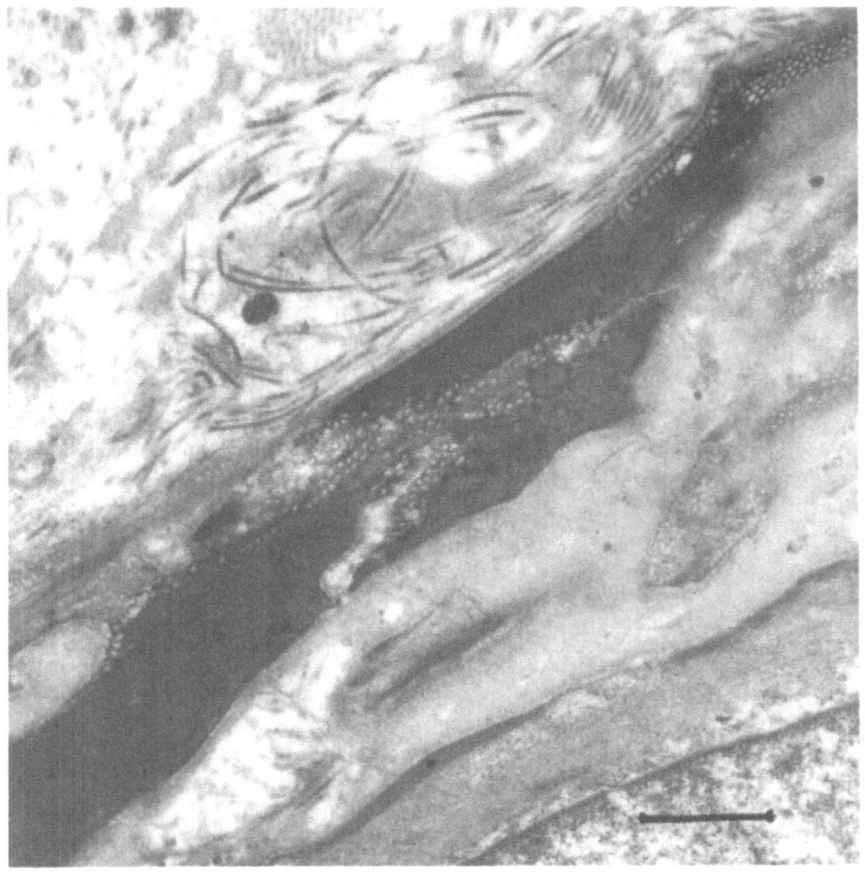

Figure 8 Necrosis of smooth muscle cells. Dense and homogenized cytoplasm, and conspicuous pinocytosis. At the bottom, normal cell. ⸺ = 1 μm

adaptation[90] of Verhoeff's iron haematoxylin show, in the early stages of the lesions, fragmentation at many points and intermingling of elastin debris and collagen fibres (initial elastolysis) (Figure 6).

(2) At a later stage, the elastic lamina disappears; between the endothelium and what remains of the media, there stretches a broad hypocellular zone occupied by material made up of two constituents: fairly abundant deteriorating collagen, and elastin debris in small lumps, some of them comma-shaped, dispersed and spilling out towards the media (final-stage elastolysis) (Figure 7).

(3) The smooth muscle cells of the media that are caught by this zone and then swallowed up show disorientation and signs of degeneration; in some cases, cell necrosis is preceded by intense pinocytosis (Figure 8).

(4) These dispersed dead cell bodies—the breakdown products of the elastin system—are significant lesions in the parenchymatous network.

These lesions begin at puberty and continue throughout the period of cyclical genital activity. Progressive reduction of the functional vascular bed seems to play a highly important role in the cessation of follicle development. For a long time afterwards, the stroma—with its diffuse vascular architecture and more regular, less perturbed flow—retains its functional potential and responds to non-cyclical LH stimulation.

References

1. Judd, H. L., Judd, G. E., Lucas, W. E. and Yen, S. S. C. (1974). Endocrine function of the postmenopausal ovary; concentration of androgens and estrogens in ovarian and peripheral vein blood. *J. Clin. Endocrinol. Metab.*, **39**, 1020–4

2. Smith, G. and Van, S. (1941). Carcinoma of endometrium. Review with results of treatment. *N. Engl. J. Med.*, **225**, 608–15

3. Fraenkel, L. (1943). Thecoma and hyperthecosis of the ovary. *J. Clin. Endocrinol. Metab.*, **3**, 557–99

4. Laffargue, P., Luscan, R. and Lavernhe, P. (1952). Hyperplasie fonctionnelle du stroma ovarien, thécome et cancer de l'endomètre. *Bull. Assoc. Fr. Cancer*, **39**, 290–305

5. Rice, B. F. and Savard, K. (1966). Steroid hormone formation in the human ovary. (IV) Ovarian stromal compartment: formation of radioactive steroids from acetate I-[14C] and action of gonadotrophins. *J. Clin. Endocrinol.*, **26**, 593–609

6. Longcope, C., Pratt, J. H., Schneider, S. H. and Fineberg, S. E. (1978). Aromatization of androgens by muscle and adipose tissue *in vivo*. *J. Clin. Endocrinol. Metab.*, **46**, 146

7. Netter, A., Mussett, R. and Poitout, Ph. (1970). Thécome ovarien associé à un adénocarcinome de l'endomètre: étude biochimique. *Bull. Fed. Soc. Gynecol. Obstet. Franç.*, **22**, 431–8

8. Vermeulen, A. (1976). The hormonal activity of the postmenopausal ovary. *J. Clin. Endocrinol. Metab.*, **42**, 247–52

9. Yen, S. S. C. (1977). The biology of menopause. *J. Reprod. Med.*, **18**, 287

10. Dennefors, B. L., Janson, P. O., Knutson, F. and Hamberger, L. (1980). Steroid production and responsiveness to gonadotropin in isolated stromal tissue of human postmenopausal ovaries. *Am. J. Obstet, Gynecol.*, **136**, 997–1002

11. Dao, T. (1953). Estrogen secretion in women with mammary cancer before and after adrenalectomy. *Science*, **118**, 21

12. Baird, D. T. (1971). Steroids in blood reflecting ovarian function. In Baird, D. T. and Strong, J. A. (eds.) *Control of Gonadal Steroid Secretion*. pp. 176–89. (Edinburgh: University Press)

13. Kirshner, M. A. and Jacobs, J. B. (1971). Combined ovarian and adrenal vein catheterization to determining the sites of androgen overproduction in hirsute women. *J. Clin. Endocrinol. Metab.*, **33**, 199–209

14. Wallart (1942). Le cortex de l'ovaire humain. *Bull. Histol. Appl. Physiol. Pathol.*, **19**, 195

15. Hertig, A. T. (1944). The ageing ovary, a preliminary note. *J. Clin. Endocrinol. Metab.*, **4**, 581

16. Bigelow, B. (1958). Comparison of ovarian and endometrial morphology spanning the menopause. *Obstet. Gynecol.*, **11**, 487

17. Fienberg, R. and Cohen, R. B. (1965). A comparative histochemical study. *Am. J. Obstet. Gynecol.*, **92**, 958–69
18. Guraya, S. S. (1966). Histochemical analysis of the interstitial gland tissue in the human ovary. *Am. J. Obstet. Gynecol.*, **96**, 907–12
19. Ryan, K. J. and Petro, Z. (1966). Steroid biosynthesis by human ovarian granulosa and theca cells. *J. Clin. Endocrinol.*, **26**, 46–52
20. Laffargue, P., Adechy-Benkoel, L. and Valette, C. (1968). Ultrastructure du stroma ovarien. *Ann. Ana-Pathol.*, **13**, 381–402
21. Laffargue, F. (1974). *Ovaire Normal et Tumeurs Endocrines de l'Ovaire. Histoenzymologie, Microscopie Electronique.* PhD Thesis, University of Marseille
22. Judd, H. L., Lucas, W. E. and Yen, S. S. C. (1976). Serum 17 beta estradiol and estrone levels in postmenopausal women with and without endometrial cancer. *J. Clin. Endocrinol. Metab.*, **43**, 272–6
23. MacNatty, K. P. (1980). The intraovarian sites of androgen and estrogen formation in women with normal and hyperandrogenic ovaries as judged by *in vitro* experiments. *J. Clin. Endocrinol. Metab.*, **50**, 755–63
24. Wehefritz, E. (1923). Systematische Gewischtsuntersuchungen am ovarien mit Berucksichtigung anderer Drusen mit innerer Sekretion. *Z. Ges. Anat.*, **9**, 161
25. Boss, J. H., Scully, R. E., Wegner, K. H. and Cohen, R. B. (1965). Structural variations in the adult ovary. Clinical significance. *J. Am. Coll. Obstet. Gynecol.*, **25**, 747–63
26. Fienberg, R. (1969). The stromal theca cell and postmenopausal adenocarcinoma. *Cancer*, **24**, 32–8
27. Bloch, E., Romney, S. L., Klein, M., Lipiello, L., Cooper, P. and Goldring, I. P. (1952). Steroid synthesis by human foetal adrenals and ovaries maintained in organic culture. *Proc. Soc. Exp. Biol.*, **119**, 449–52
28. Novak, E. R. (1970). *Obstet. Gynecol.*, **36**, 903–10
29. Scully, R. E. (1964). Stromal luteoma of the ovary. A distinctive type of lipoid-cell tumor. *Cancer*, **17**, 769–78
30. Woll, E. A. and Hertig, A. T. (1948). The ovary in endometrial carcinoma with notes on the morphological history of the aging ovary. *Am. J. Obstet. Gynecol.*, **56**, 617
31. Yen, S. C. and Jaffe, R. B. (1978). *Reproductive Endocrinology*. (Philadelphia: W. B. Saunders)
32. Giacomelli, F., Wierner, J. and Spiro, D. (1965). Cytological alterations related to stimulation of the zona glomerulosa of the adrenal gland. *J. Cell. Biol.*, **26**, 499–521
33. Deane, H. W. (1958). Intracellular lipids; their detection and significance. In Palaty, S. L. (ed.) *Frontiers in Cytology*. (New Haven: Yale University Press)
34. Fawcett, D. W. and Burgos, M. H. (1960). Studies on the fine structure of the mammalian testis. II. The human interstitial tissue. *Am. J. Anat.*, **107**, 245–69
35. Arthur, L., Christensen, F., *et al.* (1968). Localization of phosphatase in lipofuscin granules and possible autophagic vacuoles in interstitial cells of the guinea pig testis. *J. Cell. Biol.*, **36**, 1–13
36. Sato, S. (1965). An electron microscope study on the fine structure of the ovary in normal mature rats. *Arch. Histol. Jpn.*, **26**, 115–49
37. Adechy-Benkoel, L. (1973). *Etude de la Stéroidogénèse chez la Femme (Cytoenzymologie-Ultrastructure)*. Thèse Sciences, Faculté Provence, Marseille
38. Familiari, G., Franchitto, G., Correr, S. and Motta, P. (1979). Microperoxysomes in steroidogenic cells of the rat ovary; interstitial, thecal and luteal cells. *Experientia*, **35**, 1503–5
39. Loubet, R. and Loubet, A. (1961). Les cellules du hile de l'ovaire et leurs rapports avec les a tres éléments endocrines de la glande. *Ann. Anat. Pathol.*, **6**, 189–212
40. Balboni, G. C. (1976). Histology of the ovary. In James, V. H. T., Serio, M. and Giusti, G. (eds.) *The Endocrine Function of the Human Ovary*. pp. 1–24. (London: Academic Press)
41. Watenberg, L. W. (1958). Microscopic histochemical demonstration of stéroid 3 béta-ol deshydrogenase in tissue sections. *J. Histochem. Cytochem.*, **6**, 225–32
42. Botella-Llusia, J. (1980). Testosterone and 17 beta-oestradiol secretion of human ovary. *Maturitas*, **2–1**, 1–5
43. Batta, S. K. and Channing, C. P. (1979). Steroidogenesis by the various cell types of normal, cystic and postmenopausal human ovary. In Gonzales-Merloj and Giu, J. I. (eds.) *Sixth Symposio International Actualization en Obstetricia y Ginecologica, Endocrinologia, Fisiologicia, Fetal Tumares de Ovario.* (Barcelona: Salvat)
44. Corner, G. W. (1938). The sites of formation of estrogenic substances in the animal body. *Physiol. Rev.*, **18**, 154–72
45. Polyak, A., Jones, G., Goldberg, B., Solomon, D. and Woodruff, J. D. (1968). Effect of human chorionic gonadotrophin on postmenopausal women. *Am. J. Obstet. Gynecol.*, **101**, 737–9

46. MacKay, D. G. (1957). Ovarian cortical stromal hyperplasia. In Meigs, J. V. and Sturgis, S. H. (eds.) *Progress in Gynecology*. Vol. III. (New York: Grune and Stratton)
47. Kondtsaal, J., Bossenbrock, B. and Hardonk, M. J. (1968). Ovarian tumors investigated by histochemical and enzyme histochemical methods. *Am. J. Obstet. Gynecol.*, 102, 1004–77
48. Geller, S., Ayme, Y., Kandelman, M., Grisoli, F., Lemasson, C. and Scholler, R. (1975). Ovaires polykystiques. Secrétion inappropriée de L.H. 'seule'. Microadénome à L.H.? *N. Press. Méd.*, 5, 1492
49. Pfleiderer, A. and Teufel, G. (1968). Incidence and histochemical investigation of enzymatically active cells in stroma of ovarian tumors. *Am. J. Obstet. Gynecol.*, 102, 997–1003
50. Tait, J. F. and Burstein, S. (1964). *In vivo* studies of steroid dynamics in man. In Pinkus, G. (ed.) *The Hormones*. pp. 441–55. (New York: Academic Press)
51. Rivarola, A. M., Saez, J., Jones, H. W., Jone, J. G. and Migeon, Cl. (1967). The secretion of androgens by the normal polycystic and neoplastic ovaries. *Johns Hopkins Med. J.*, 121, 82
52. Mattingly, R. and Huang, W. Y. (1969). Steroidogenesis of the menopausal and post-menopausal ovary. *Am. J. Obstet. Gynecol.*, 103, 679
53. Jong, F. H., Baird, D. T. and van der Molen, H. S. (1974). *Acta Endocrinol.*, 77, 575–87. Quoted in James, V. H. T., Serio, M. and Giusti, G. (eds.) *The Endocrine Function of the Human Ovary* (1976). (London: Academic Press)
54. Rader, M. D., Flikinger, G. L., de Villa, G. O., Jr., Mikuta, J. J. and Mikhail, G. (1973). Plasma estrogens in postmenopausal women. *Am. J. Obstet. Gynecol.*, 116, 1069–73
55. Mahesh, V. B. and Greenblatt, R. B. (1964). Steroid secretions of the normal and polycystic ovary. *Rec. Prog. Horm. Res.*, 21, 341–94
56. Givens, J. R., Wiser, W. L., Coleman, S. A., Wilroy, R. S., Anderson, R. N. and Fish, S. A. (1971). Familial ovarian hyperthecosis, study of two families. *Am. J. Obstet. Gynecol.*, 110, 959–72
57. Mauvais-Jarvis, P. and Bercovici, J-P. (1968). Biogénèse des stéroides ovariens. *Press. Méd.*, 76, 571–4
58. Mauvais-Jarvis, P. and Bercovici, J-P. (1968). Sécretion, production et interconversion des principaux androgènes (sujets normaux et femmes hirsutes). *Press. Méd.*, 76, 1767–70
59. Jones, G. E. S., Goldberg, J. D. and Woodruff, J. D. (1968). Cell specific steroid inhibitions in histochemical stéroid 3 beta-ol deshydrogenase activities in man. *Histochimica*, 14, 131–42
60. Laffargue, P., Smadja, A., Nony, Y. and Audrin, N. (1969). Répliques dysplasiques des tumeurs endocrines de l'ovaire. *Arch. Ana-Pathol.*, 17, A 202–4
61. Clinton, C. W., Rogaly, E. and Bernstein (1981). Leydig–Sertoli cell tumour in a post-menopausal female. *S. Afr. Med. J.*, 434–5
62. Morris, J. Mc. and Scully, R. E. (1958). *Endocrine Pathology of the Ovary*. pp. 131–9. (St Louis: C. V. Mosby)
63. Si Chun Ming, M. D. and Golman, H. (1962). Hormonal activity of Brenner tumors in post-menopausal woman. *Am. J. Obstet. Gynecol.*, 83, 666–73
64. Woodruff, J. D., Goldberg, B. and Jones, G. E. S. (1968). Enzymic histochemical reactions in two Krukenberg tumors associated with clinically different endocrine patterns. *Am. J. Obstet. Gynecol.*, 100, 405–17
65. Fox, H. (1965). Estrogenic activity of the serous cystadenoma of the ovary. *Cancer*, 18, 1041–7
66. Eddie, D. A. S. (1967). Ovarian stromal response to neoplasia and the relationship with hormone production. *J. Obstet. Gynaecol. Br. Commonw.*, 74, 286–91
67. Edwards, R. L., Nicholson, H. O., Zoidis, T., Bott, W. R. and Taylor, C. W. (1971). Endocrine studies in postmenopausal women with ovarian tumors. *J. Obstet. Gynaecol. Br. Commonw.*, 78, 467–77
68. Edman, C. D. and MacDonald, P. S. (1976). The role of extraglandular estrogen in women in health and disease. In James, V. H. T., Serio, M. and Giusti, G. (eds.) *The Endocrine Function of the Human Ovary*. pp. 135–40. (London: Academic Press)
69. Hamwi, G. J., Byron, R. C., Besch, P. G., Vorys, N., Teteris, N. J. and Uller, J. C. (1963). Testosterone synthesis by a Brenner tumor. Clinical evidence of masculinization during pregnancy. *Am. J. Obstet. Gynecol.*, 86, 1015–20
70. Meiling, R. L., Boutselis, J. G., Teteris, N. J., Ullery, J. C. and Georges, O. T. (1963). Histochemical observations on a Brenner cell tumor with masculinization. *Am. J. Obstet. Gynecol.*, 87, 463–70
71. Scully, R. E. and Cohen, R. B. (1964). Oxidative enzyme activity in normal and pathologic human ovaries. *Obstet. Gynecol.*, 24, 667–80
72. Janovski, N. A. and Paramanandhan (1970). Enzymatically active stromal nature of the Reinke cristalloide. *Obstet. Gynecol.*, 35, 493–503

73. Rome, R. M. and Laverty, C. R. (1973). Ovarian tumours in postmenopausal women. *J. Obstet. Gynaecol. Br. Commonw.*, **80**, 984–91
74. Langley, F. A. and Fox, H. (1978). Tumeurs endocrines de l'ovaire. In Scholler, R. (ed.) *Endocrinologie de l'Ovaire*. (Paris: SEPE)
75. Hughesdon, P. E. (1958). Thecal and allied reactions in epithelial ovarian tumours. *J. Obstet. Gynaecol. Br. Emp.*, **63**, 702–9
76. Brux, J. de (1971). *Histopathologie Gynécologique*. Vol. 1. *Collection d'Histopathologie*. (Paris: Masson)
77. Greenblatt, R. B. (1976). Estrogens and endometrial cancer. In Beard, R. J. (ed.) *The Menopause*. (Lancaster: MTP)
78. Somerhausen, M. and Gompel, C. (1960). Hyperplasie du stroma cortical de l'ovaire et cancer du sein. *Bull. Soc. Belg. Gynecol. Obstet.*, **30**, 467–80
79. Grodin, J. M., Siiteri, P. K. and MacDonald, P. C. (1973). Source of estrogen production in postmenopausal women. *J. Clin. Endocrinol. Metab.*, **36**, 207
80. Lipsett, M. B., Wilson, H., Kirshner, M. A., *et al.* (1966). Studies on Leydig cell physiology and pathology: secretion and metabolism of testosterone. *Rec. Prog. Horm. Res.*, **22**, 245–81
81. Brozek, J. (1961). Body composition: the relative amounts of fat tissue and water vary with age, sex, exercise and nutritional state. *Science*, **134**, 920–30
82. Rizkallah, T. H., Tovell, H. M. M. and Kelly, W. G. (1975). Production of estrone and fractional conversion of circulating androstenedione to estrone in women with endometrial carcinoma. *J. Clin. Endocrinol. Metab.*, **40**, 1045–56
83. Cedard, L., Alsat, E., Urtasun, M. J. and Varangot, J. (1970). Studies on the mode of action of luteinizing hormone and chorionic gonadotropin on estrogenic biosynthesis and glycogenolysis by human placenta perfused *in vitro*. *Steroids*, **16**, 361–75
84. Marsh, J. M. (1975). The role of cyclic AMP in gonadal function. *Adv. Cycl. Nucl. Res.*, **6**, 137–99
85. Gautray, J. P. (1968). *Reproduction Humaine*. Vol. 1, p. 22. (Paris: Masson)
86. Bellman, S., Block, E. and Odeblad, E. (1953). Microangiographic study of the minute ovarian blood vessels in albino rats. *Br. J. Radiol.*, **26**, 584–8
87. Reynolds, S. R. M. (1950). The vasculature of the ovary and ovarian function. In Pinkus, G. (ed.) *Recent Progress in Hormone Research*. Vol. 5, pp. 65–100. (New York: Academic Press)
88. Loubet, A., Loubet, R. and Leboutet, M-J. (1979). Elastolyse artérielle et sénescence ovarienne. *Gynécologie*, **30**, 133–9
89. Baird, D. T. (1974). Prostaglandin F_2 alpha and ovarian blood flow in sheep. *J. Endocrinol.*, **62**, 413–14
90. Brissie, R. M., Spicer, S. S., Hall, B. J. and Thomson, N. T. (1974). Ultrastructural staining of thin sections with ironhematoxylin. *J. Histochem. Cytochem.*, **22**, 895–907

10
Ovary and pregnancy

F. Cabanne

Associating the two words 'ovary' and 'pregnancy' suggests, at first sight, the *corpus luteum of pregnancy*, with its structure and morphological or functional history as a temporary endocrine gland, i.e. normal phenomena whose anatomy and physiology we are understanding better all the time.

Yet besides these major transformations undergone by the corpus luteum during pregnancy, the ovary also goes through *sub-normal or pathological changes*. These are varied and their significance is a matter for debate. Most of them are poorly understood. It is our intention to discuss the most frequent.

SUB-NORMAL OVARIAN LESIONS

Stromal *oedema and congestion* are incidental findings which are almost never marked. It is the medulla that is particularly affected. Oedema and congestion are associated with marked dilatation of the hilar vessels, and they occur with a frequency that is impossible to determine.

Luteinization of ovarian stroma cells may be considered as being at the limits of normal physiology. Small clumps of round or elongated cells are affected, which stand out clearly against the other stromal cells because of their clear, pale cytoplasm (Figure 1). These clumps are spread throughout the ovary containing the corpus luteum, or even in the contralateral ovary. Luteinization may also touch, to a slight degree, the granulosa or theca cells of the other follicles in the ovary, even if these follicles are old or regressing. These events have no clinical repercussions and are dependent on placental FSH, LH and chorionic gonadotrophin secretion.

LUTEINIZED THECAL CYST

This is also known as 'luteinized granulosa theca cyst', an expression which gives a perfect idea of its histogenesis.

This cyst has a pale core and a thick wall made of large hypertrophied theca cells and small granulosa cells which are occasionally atrophied. It is surrounded by ovarian stroma as well as by some non-cystic follicles which show signs of marked pro-gestational metaplasia (Figure 2).

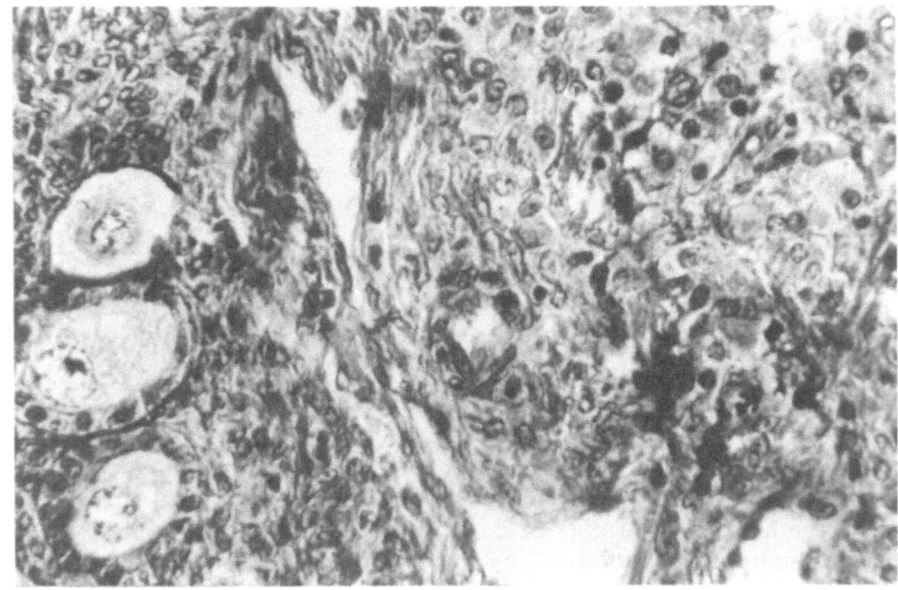

Figure 1 Ovarian stroma cell luteinization in a woman aged 23. Note the round cells with clear cytoplasm. Note also, on the left, three primordial follicles surrounded by granulosa cells   (× 250)

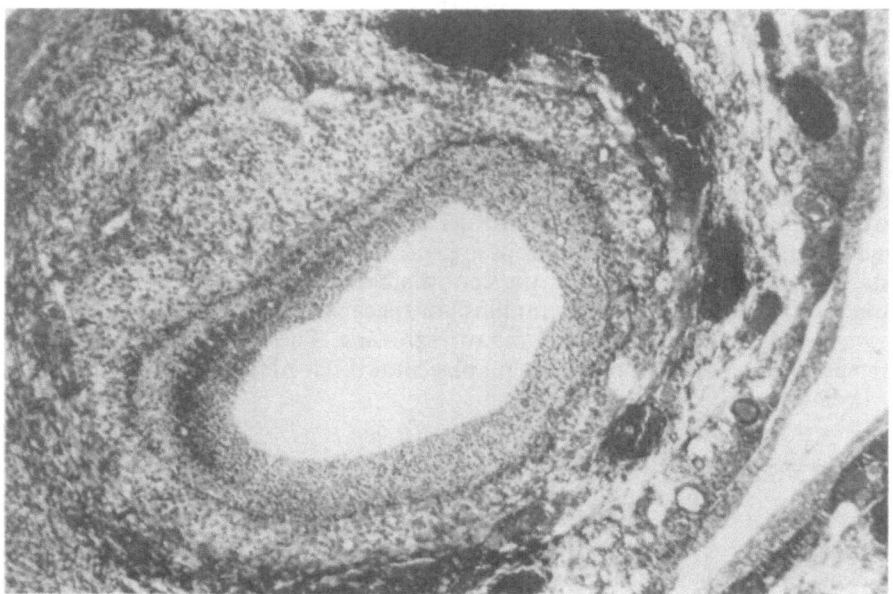

Figure 2 Luteinized thecal cyst in a woman aged 28. Note the double wall, with the inner thin layer of granulosa and the outer thick layer of luteinized theca cells   (× 27)

These cysts are bulky, and may be multiple or bilateral. To the naked eye, they are bright yellow on section, with haemorrhagic spots and streaks.

LH and FSH hyperstimulation causes the lesion, spontaneous regression of which takes place when the original hormone source dries up. This is why such cysts can always be found in the course of hydatidiform mole, less frequently in cases of choriocarcinoma and occasionally even in a so-called 'normal' pregnancy.

'LUTEOMA OF PREGNANCY'

This is the expression coined by Sternberg and Barclay, in their description of a lesion which is not a tumour in the strict sense. It consists essentially in a massive and pseudo-tumoural luteinization of ovarian stroma cells. Luteinized thecal cysts are also quite often found. This association helps to explain why gestational luteoma is sometimes all solid, and sometimes half-cystic, half-solid (Figure 3).

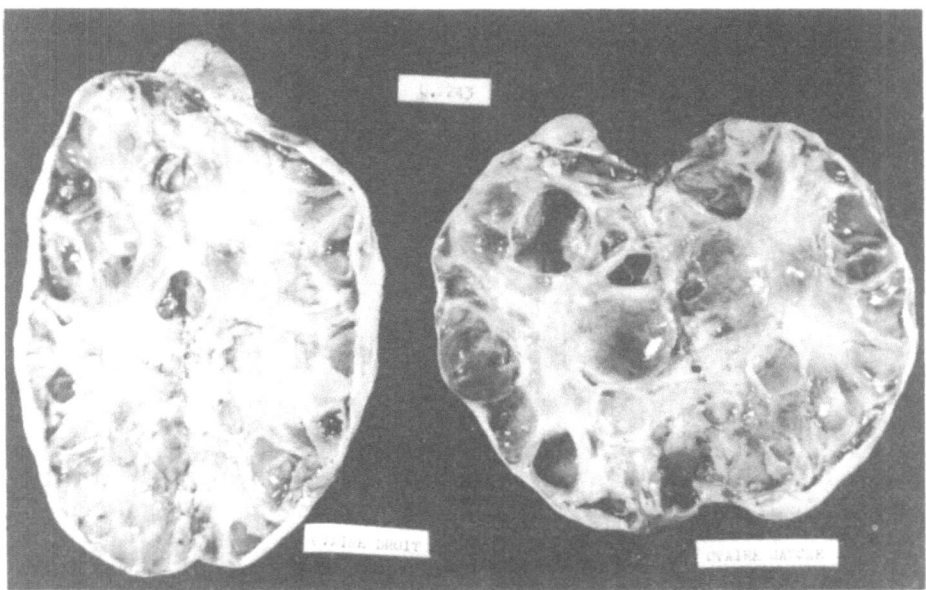

Figure 3   Bilateral luteoma of pregnancy in a woman aged 23 (half-cystic, half-solid)

The luteoma is bilateral in 50% of cases. It can develop in conjunction with an ovarian tumour such as a mucinous cystadenoma.

The tumour-like hyperplasia, as it has been called, is capable of producing oestrogens, progesterone, or androgens. It can be responsible for a virilization syndrome in the mother or fetus (if a female).

Gestational luteoma is in fact an exaggeration of the process mentioned above. It corresponds to excessive response to gonadotrophin action. This is, incidentally, the reason why it appears during pregnancy and spontaneously disappears after delivery.

CYSTIC AND HAEMORRHAGIC CORPUS LUTEUM

This lesion is due to extreme hyperplasia of the functional corpus luteum, the centre of which consists of a cavity being gradually distended by sero-haemorrhagic fluid. The luteal cells surrounding the cavity appear hypertrophied (Figure 4).

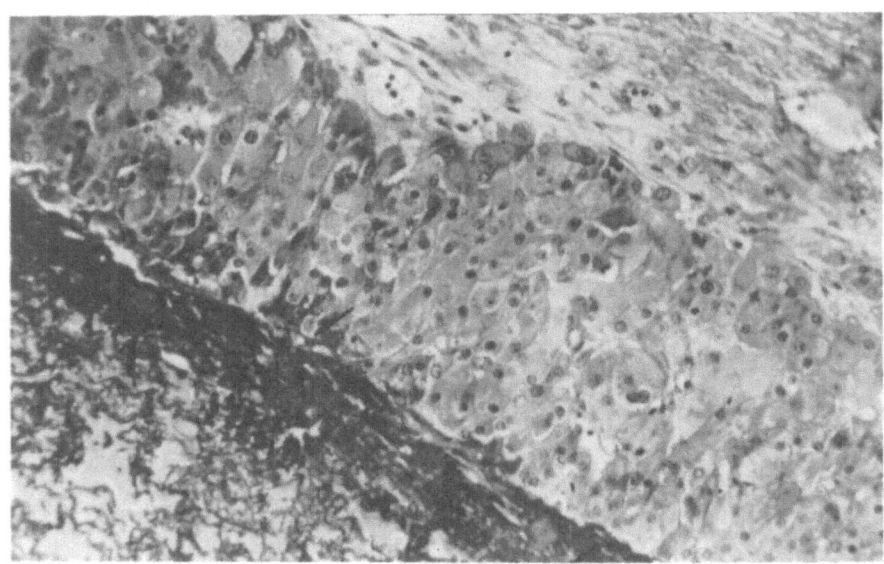

Figure 4 Cystic and haemorrhagic corpus luteum in a woman aged 25. Note the layer of hypertrophied luteal cells, surrounding a fibro-haemorrhagic area, on the left and below (× 114)

The yellow body of the cyst may be seen with the naked eye bulging from the surface of the ovary. Its presence is known to account for pelvic pain of varying degrees. The cyst is also known to rupture and be responsible for intra-peritoneal haemorrhage, giving a misleading acute abdominal syndrome, mimicking the rupture of an ectopic pregnancy.

This abnormality affects the pro-gestational, rather than the gestational body, and its pathogenesis is still unknown.

OVARIAN DECIDUOSIS

The main feature of this condition is the presence of small islands of large, clear decidual cells in the ovarian cortex and, occasionally, in the medulla. The cells are identical with those in normal pregnancy decidua (Figure 5). They remain side by side, without a hint of developing glandular structure. Collagen fibres often traverse these islands, which are infiltrated by fibro-hyaline deposit. The boundary separating them from neighbouring ovarian stroma is frequently imprecise.

With the naked eye, masses of ovarian deciduosis can be seen as pinkish-grey spots reminiscent of tuberculous granulation. They are as a rule multiple and bilateral.

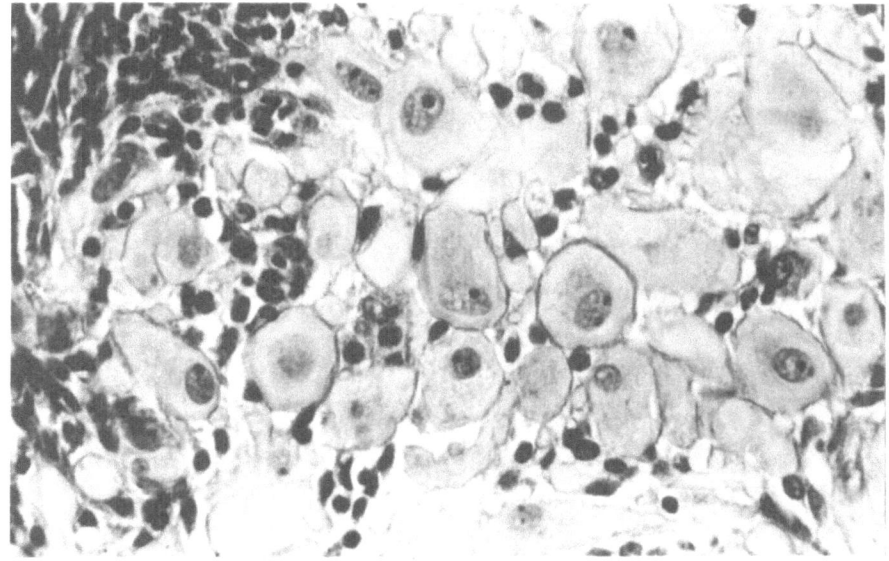

Figure 5 Ovarian deciduosis with large cells, side by side, in a woman aged 29. Note the clear cytoplasm, the large nucleus and the obvious nucleolus (× 304)

Ovarian deciduosis appears during the first trimester of pregnancy, develops, then spontaneously disappears post-partum. Its frequency is difficult to determine. Most probably it is high, since deciduosis affects most of the ovaries that are removed during pregnancy and can often be seen around ovarian tumours occurring during gestation. It naturally reshapes foci of ovarian endometriosis and can disrupt them in such a way that they disappear post-partum.

Ovarian deciduosis most probably corresponds, like other ectopic deciduomas (of the cervix or pelvic peritoneum, for example), to metaplasia of sensitive mesenchymatous tissues, such as cytogenous chorion, under the hormonal stimuli of pregnancy.

OVARIAN PREGNANCY

This condition is mentioned here more for the sake of completeness than to state new facts.

The diagnosis of primary ovarian pregnancy can be made only in the presence of a yolk sac or fragments of embryo in the middle of a corpus luteum partially destroyed by trophoblastic villosities. Masses of decidual cells are scattered all over the congested and haemorrhagic ovarian tissue which remains in the periphery. This type of ovarian pregnancy is rare and makes up only 1% of all ectopic pregnancies.

Fimbrio-ovarian pregnancy, caused by adhesions between the fimbriae and the ovary, goes beyond the scope of this study. The ovum is para-ovarian. Strictly speaking, the ovarian parenchyma becomes dissociated only by haemorrhagic foci containing trophoblastic villosities and by islands of deciduoma.

Finally, it is interesting to note that apart from ovarian pregnancy, all ovarian changes are an expression of hormone stimulation and a response by gonadal cells. Thus during pregnancy the ovary appears to be an endocrine gland, producing oestrogens and progesterone, as well as being a 'hormone receptor'.

IV—Clinical Physiopathology

11
Clinical investigation of luteal defect: a model for understanding the endocrine correlates of the menstrual cycle disorders

J.-P. Gautray, D. Rotten, J. C. Thalabard, J. P. Vielh, M. C. Colin, K. Nahoul and J. de Brux

Toutes les fois où l'on prétendra présenter
un travail complet où rien ne reste absent,
on pourra dire que celà est faux.

Claude Bernard

Although Wentz noticed the higher frequency of articles on luteal defect (LD)[1], the effects of this disorder, its influence on fecundity, its physiopathology, and its therapy are still uncertain and debated. Following Jones[2–4], we have used endometrial biopsy (EB) as the reference criterion for investigation of LD. Two different patterns of the progesterone insufficient influence on the endometrium have been previously described: the first is a delay or a lack of progesterone effect which induces an *out of phase endometrium* (Figure 1(*a*) and (*b*)), while a persistent oestrogenic influence (PEI) is associated to luteal defect in the second pattern, as if progesterone effect was too weak to blunt the oestrogenic one (Figure 1(*c*) and (*d*)). These endometrial patterns were correlated to ovarian steroid plasma values[5].

The prospect of this study was to investigate the gonadotrophins and prolactin balance in LD which was clinically suspected, but ascertained by EB. The results have led to a better understanding of the physiopathology of this functional gynaecological disorder which often induces infecundity. Consequently, a rationale for the clinical investigation of the menstrual cycle is proposed. LD may be the terminal expression of different mechanisms and/or endocrine disorders. The proposed method of investigation should help to differentiate groups of patients according to the pathogenesis of LD.

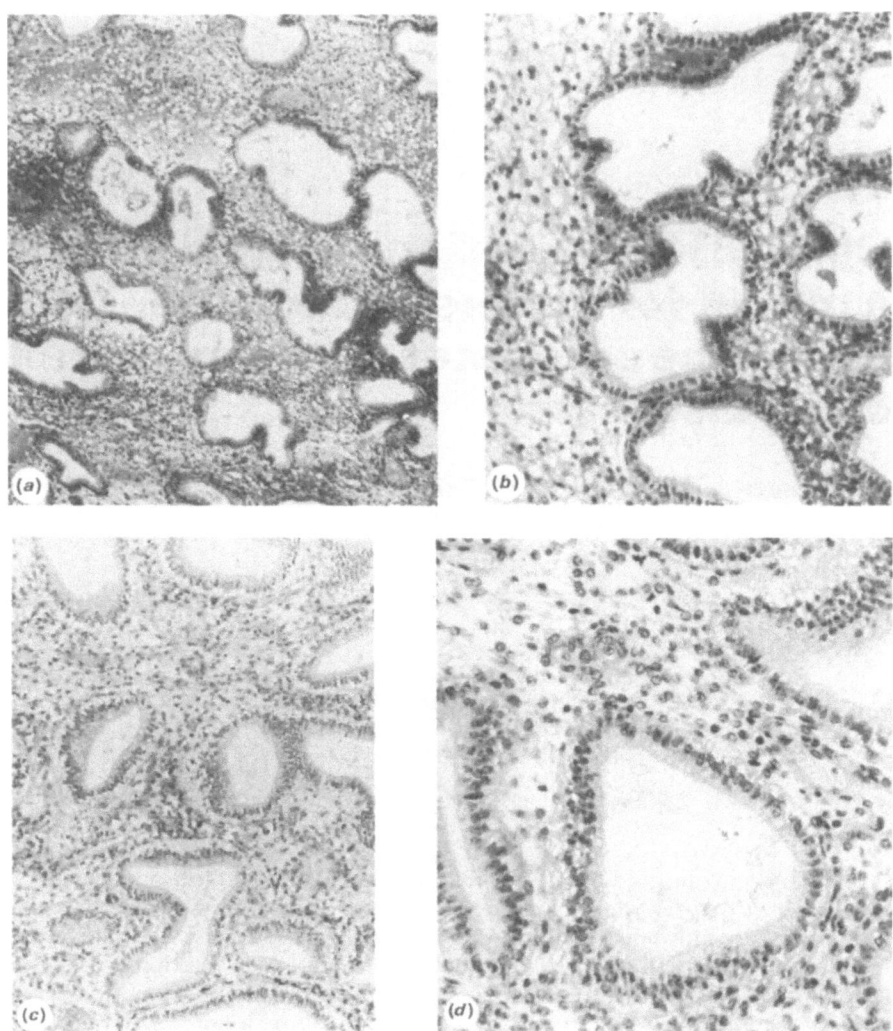

Figure 1   (a) and (b) Endometrial histological definition of pure luteal defect, on day 23. The stroma is oedematous, the glandular tubes are dilated, only slightly wavy, connective spines are scarce, the glandular secretion is poor; very similar to day 19 ($a \times 80$; $b \times 200$). (c) and (d) Luteal defect plus persistent oestrogenic influence, on day 25. The stroma is dense and its cellularity is high, the tubes are dilated, regular or scarcely wavy, multistratification and mitosis are still obvious and secretion is poor; very similar to day 16 ($c \times 80$; $d \times 200$)

PLASMA CONCENTRATION OF GONADOTROPHINS

Many reports have recently demonstrated the role of FSH, and its relation to LH in follicle development, granulosa cell maturation and oestradiol secretion. Ovulation, corpus luteum and endometrium adequacy are dependent on these physiological events. However, longitudinal studies of FSH, LH levels, and

FSH:LH ratios are scarce in humans[6]. Plasma FSH and LH levels have been investigated and correlated with the usual criteria of LD, and compared with normal cycles.

Materials and methods

Fifteen patients were investigated in the Gynaecology Department Outpatient Clinic. They all complained of infertility. The investigation included basal body temperature (BBT) charts, an EB and daily plasma hormone measurements throughout the whole menstrual cycle.

BBT charts were performed during at least three cycles. The lowest point before the temperature rise was considered as the presumed ovulation date. Although the BBT chart only reflects the thermogenic influence of progesterone, it is nevertheless considered as a valuable tool for an initial clinical approach. The length of each phase was estimated in days, a previous statistical study of normal cycles having demonstrated the value of this investigation[7]. Luteal defect cannot be ascertained on BBT charts only, but can be suspected if recurrent short luteal phases of less than 10 days' duration are observed, or if basal temperature is not stable during the same period[5].

EB was performed between day 21 and day 23, during the possible implantation period, when endometrial transformations are at their best. Later on, the histological modifications preceding menstruation will appear[8,9]. EB ascertains the suspected luteal defect[5,8] (Figure 1).

Blood samples were collected on dry tubes (20 ml), every day of these 15 cycles, at the same time for each patient, the first one being taken on the first day of menstruation. Decantation, centrifugation and freezing at $-20°C$ allowed preservation of samples until radioimmunoassays for LH, FSH, oestradiol-17β (E_2), progesterone (P) and 17α-OHP were carried out[10-12].

The results have been compared with 27 control cycles where LH peak, luteal phase length and progesterone levels were considered as normal. These control investigations had been previously performed (Fondation de Recherche en Hormonologie). For each hormone, each day mean value of the control cycles was calculated and plotted on a curve, with the extreme values. This curve was considered as normal, and used for comparison for each daily hormonal value of the investigated cycles. FSH:LH ratio was calculated every day for each patient and compared also with the values obtained in the control cycles.

Results

Daily plasma hormone concentrations are displayed in Tables 1 and 2. Investigative attention was focused on the first week of the cycle, on behalf of previous experimental studies[14,19-23], and of course on the luteal phase. The FSH:LH ratio was used as a discriminant tool to classify these patients (Figure 2). A first group (group I), of nine patients (Table 1, Figures 2 and 3) is characterized by a slight lowering of the FSH:LH ratio during the first week of the cycle. However, the ratio values are quite similar to the mean value of the control group during the other parts of the cycle. A second group (group II), of six patients is characterized by a very low FSH:LH ratio (Table 2, Figures 2 and 4). Using the Wilcoxon non-parametric test, statistically significant differences of LH values and FSH:LH ratios could be observed on days -14 to -7, between those two groups of patients ($p < 0.01$).

Table 1 FSH:LH ratio, FSH, LH, oestradiol (E_2), progesterone (P) and 17α-OHP values (as means, with SE in parentheses) in the nine patients characterized by a decrease of FSH:LH ratio during the first week of the cycle

Hormone	−14	−13	−12	−11	−10	−9	−8	−7	−6	−5	−4	−3	−2	−1
FSH:LH	2.57 (0.65)	1.88 (0.37)	1.92 (0.30)	1.70 (0.37)	1.61 (0.37)	1.75 (0.44)	1.64 (0.42)	1.52 (0.45)	1.49 (0.46)	1.33 (0.47)	1.19 (0.41)	1.05 (0.29)	1.03 (0.40)	0.74 (0.31)
FSH mIU/ml	6.93 (3.11)	4.70 (0.93)	5.07 (1.39)	4.23 (1.43)	4.62 (0.87)	4.99 (2.19)	4.83 (1.20)	4.61 (1.22)	4.26 (0.52)	4.16 (1.10)	3.81 (0.94)	3.41 (1.07)	3.33 (1.23)	3.47 (1.64)
LH mIU/ml	2.68 (0.73)	2.52 (0.36)	2.77 (1.13)	2.84 (0.86)	2.97 (0.75)	2.91 (0.89)	3.10 (1.06)	3.30 (1.36)	3.13 (1.17)	3.43 (1.34)	3.52 (1.29)	3.40 (1.14)	3.33 (0.63)	5.27 (2.91)
E_2 pg/ml	44.75 (17.35)	48.40 (16.64)	47.33 (18.00)	55.88 (21.66)	47.78 (17.95)	61.33 (28.67)	69.67 (35.21)	83.44 (69.00)	157.00 (260.58)	126.33 (107.70)	166.11 (174.04)	226.33 (246.65)	302.78 (377.40)	332.00 (302.88)
P ng/ml													0.04 (0.00)	0.04 (0.00)
17α-OHP ng/ml	0.22 (0.21)	0.30 (0.25)	0.18 (0.21)	0.25 (0.22)	0.21 (0.22)	0.21 (0.20)	0.26 (0.28)	0.49 (0.52)	0.40 (0.35)	0.32 (0.33)	0.46 (0.48)	0.48 (0.64)	0.59 (0.72)	0.64 (0.47)

Hormone	0	1	2	3	4	5	6	7	8	9	10	11	12	13
FSH:LH	0.37 (0.14)	0.72 (0.38)	1.02 (0.45)	1.20 (0.49)	1.11 (0.62)	1.08 (0.68)	1.22 (0.72)	1.17 (0.61)	0.93 (0.53)	0.94 (0.66)	1.17 (0.65)	0.97 (0.44)	1.11 (0.53)	1.08 (0.39)
FSH mIU/ml	8.67 (5.10)	6.69 (5.67)	4.09 (1.56)	3.57 (1.27)	3.09 (1.20)	2.96 (0.79)	2.73 (1.09)	2.56 (0.96)	1.98 (0.81)	1.98 (0.93)	1.73 (0.81)	1.69 (0.62)	1.64 (0.26)	2.00 (0.38)
LH mIU/ml	25.48 (17.59)	10.52 (7.91)	4.60 (2.37)	3.30 (1.71)	3.47 (2.38)	4.31 (3.47)	2.66 (1.14)	2.76 (1.87)	2.48 (1.44)	2.66 (1.19)	1.43 (0.48)	2.04 (1.23)	1.70 (0.67)	2.28 (1.69)
E_2 pg/ml	409.78 (469.55)	223.89 (274.88)	107.33 (73.01)	109.22 (55.14)	137.22 (99.21)	164.44 (126.32)	175.67 (114.50)	165.33 (65.15)	147.22 (42.72)	137.63 (58.74)	130.29 (49.06)	133.86 (71.60)	136.14 (57.60)	84.60 (26.66)
P ng/ml	0.45 (0.52)	1.24 (1.02)	2.46 (1.50)	5.64 (2.34)	8.22 (6.14)	8.64 (3.12)	10.56 (4.95)	10.69 (2.35)	10.88 (4.84)	10.26 (6.89)	7.99 (4.19)	5.61 (3.60)	5.40 (3.50)	2.42 (1.05)
17α-OHP ng/ml	1.90 (1.87)	1.75 (1.74)	1.56 (1.21)	2.12 (2.36)	2.23 (1.94)	2.52 (2.73)	2.52 (1.58)	2.51 (1.24)	1.90 (1.13)	1.72 (1.34)	1.68 (1.05)	1.28 (1.11)	0.88 (0.69)	0.54 (0.17)

154

Table 2 FSH:LH ratio, FSH, LH, oestradiol (E$_2$), progesterone (P) and 17α-OHP values (as means, with SE in parentheses) in the six patients characterized by a very low FSH:LH ratio

Hormone	Day													
	−14	−13	−12	−11	−10	−9	−8	−7	−6	−5	−4	−3	−2	−1
FSH:LH	1.24 (0.27)	0.89 (0.34)	1.04 (0.25)	1.00 (0.31)	0.90 (0.19)	0.93 (0.31)	1.10 (0.19)	0.80 (0.31)	0.92 (0.36)	0.73 (0.22)	0.69 (0.34)	0.71 (0.14)	0.59 (0.07)	0.35 (0.18)
FSH mIU/ml	3.82 (0.76)	3.83 (1.03)	4.93 (0.43)	4.47 (1.33)	4.45 (0.75)	4.57 (1.03)	4.32 (1.19)	4.17 (0.83)	3.83 (0.92)	3.92 (1.14)	3.20 (0.86)	2.98 (0.73)	3.62 (1.30)	5.47 (4.77)
LH mIU/ml	3.48 (0.65)	4.78 (1.11)	4.87 (0.83)	4.58 (0.86)	5.05 (0.73)	5.23 (1.61)	4.85 (1.18)	5.20 (0.84)	4.92 (2.06)	4.92 (0.86)	4.30 (0.98)	4.20 (1.56)	5.43 (1.67)	11.50 (3.62)
E$_2$ pg/ml	53.60 (34.77)	50.33 (20.56)	63.83 (37.03)	54.80 (26.62)	64.17 (33.87)	68.67 (16.82)	62.83 (20.89)	77.67 (29.10)	72.00 (14.38)	97.50 (16.13)	111.67 (32.00)	216.33 (63.83)	217.67 (52.86)	276.00 (52.99)
P ng/ml													0.04 (0.00)	0.09 (0.08)
17α-OHP ng/ml	0.49 (0.34)	0.41 (0.26)	0.44 (0.32)	0.32 (0.18)	0.37 (0.22)	0.44 (0.28)	0.47 (0.30)	0.41 (0.22)	0.39 (0.24)	0.36 (0.18)	0.34 (0.17)	0.39 (0.25)	0.44 (0.34)	0.71 (0.40)

Hormone	Day													
	0	1	2	3	4	5	6	7	8	9	10	11	12	13
FSH:LH	0.30 (0.09)	0.50 (0.27)	0.67 (0.59)	0.59 (0.31)	0.63 (0.41)	0.88 (0.66)	0.65 (0.30)	0.71 (0.34)	0.92 (0.43)	0.85 (0.68)	0.60 (0.45)	0.56 (0.38)	1.01 (0.53)	0.81 (0.31)
FSH mIU/ml	10.22 (6.09)	5.13 (1.90)	4.10 (1.45)	3.48 (1.39)	3.92 (2.05)	2.68 (1.00)	2.53 (0.73)	2.55 (0.59)	2.23 (0.55)	1.83 (0.80)	2.30 (1.29)	1.62 (0.80)	2.03 (1.43)	2.80 (1.61)
LH mIU/ml	25.95 (8.87)	9.80 (4.06)	6.63 (2.75)	5.37 (2.31)	5.88 (2.21)	3.85 (3.81)	4.42 (2.08)	3.67 (1.61)	3.05 (2.31)	2.83 (1.94)	3.92 (1.75)	2.96 (1.53)	2.17 (1.94)	3.37 (1.63)
E$_2$ pg/ml	236.50 (95.94)	133.17 (74.86)	116.17 (38.34)	121.33 (41.19)	146.67 (65.40)	161.17 (35.53)	170.17 (66.89)	180.67 (48.84)	168.67 (37.88)	142.80 (73.02)	173.20 (75.29)	193.60 (41.63)	143.33 (34.02)	198.33 (99.81)
P ng/ml	0.30 (0.22)	0.75 (0.81)	1.49 (0.95)	3.65 (1.23)	5.62 (2.20)	7.15 (3.80)	6.67 (2.40)	8.12 (4.20)	7.53 (4.47)	6.58 (4.89)	7.27 (6.03)	7.02 (6.41)	3.70 (1.65)	3.35 (3.49)
17α-OHP ng/ml	1.27 (0.35)	0.92 (0.16)	1.23 (0.30)	1.48 (0.64)	1.53 (0.79)	1.65 (0.70)	2.02 (1.37)	1.78 (1.04)	1.95 (1.20)	1.58 (0.96)	1.58 (1.10)	1.48 (0.88)	0.77 (0.12)	1.27 (0.76)

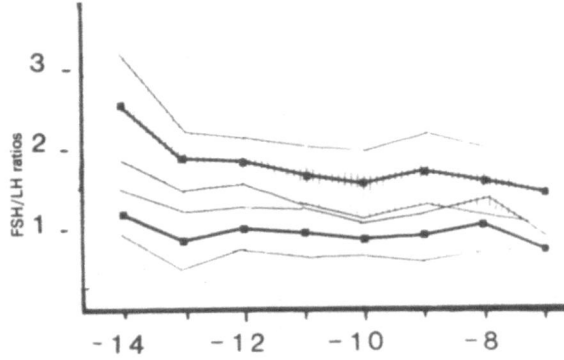

Figure 2 Development of FSH : LH ratios during the first week of 15 cycles which were synchronized acording to the LH peak (mean and SE). This histogram shows two groups of patients. The higher curve (group I, nine patients) shows a light decrease of FSH : LH ratio; the lower curve a more severe one (group II, six patients)

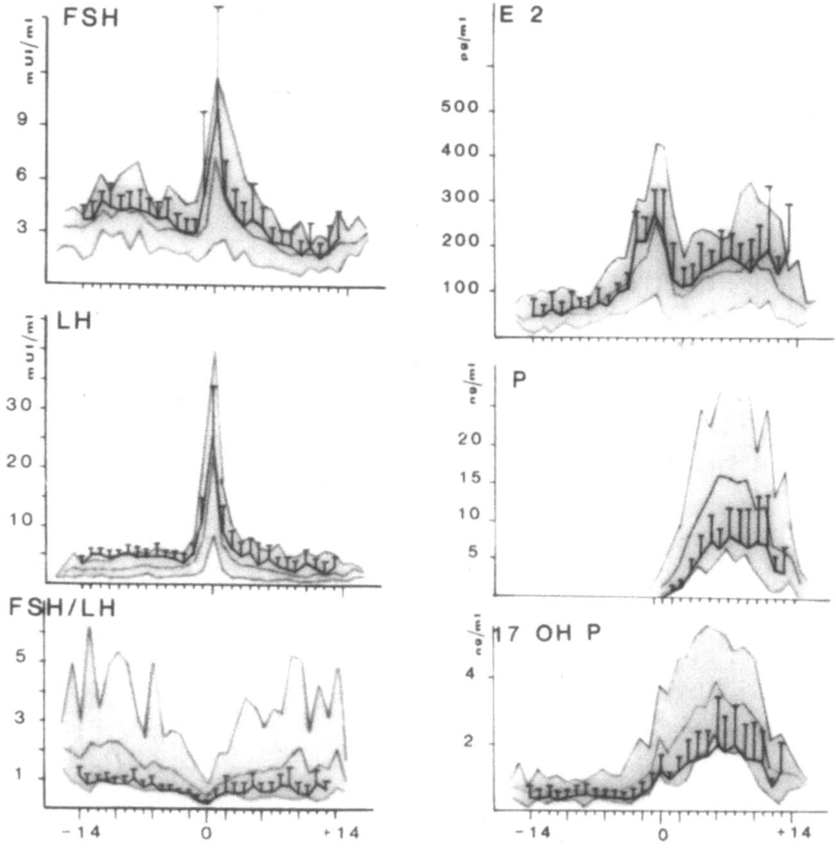

Figure 3 Plasma daily hormone concentrations and FSH : LH ratio in group I. The shaded area corresponds to the normal distribution of values during 27 control cycles. E2 = oestradiol; P = progesterone

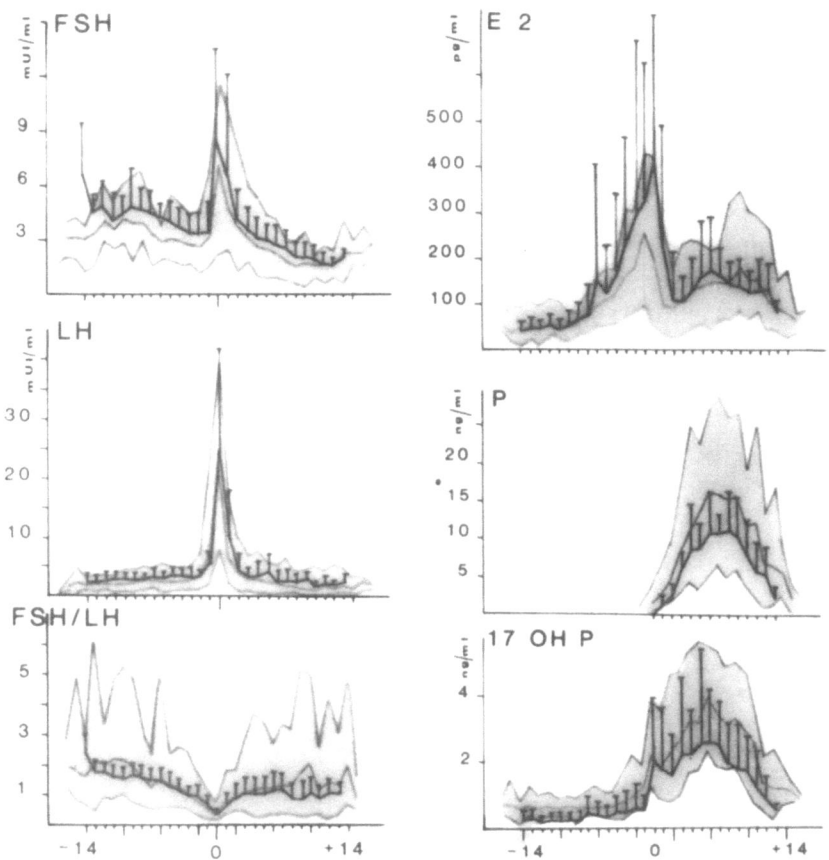

Figure 4 Daily hormone concentrations and FSH:LH ratio in group II. The shaded area corresponds to the normal distribution of values during 27 control cycles. E2 = oestradiol; P = progesterone

In the first group, LH values were approximately normal, the FSH ones were close to the values of the control group; however, the FSH decrease during the preovulatory period is not as obvious as it is in the control group. A moderate deficiency of both E_2 and P during the luteal phase was observed. The E_2 preovulatory peak was wider than usual. The endometrial biopsy of these patients demonstrated LD with PEI in six cases, and pure LD in the three others.

In the second group of six patients, mean FSH and LH values are higher than in the control group, particularly during the luteal phase. If the FSH values are approximatively at the same level in both groups, LH is obviously higher in group II. There was a statistically significant difference of daily LH values of groups I and II: (i) from days $- 13$ to $- 6$ ($p < 0.01$); (ii) $- 2$ ($p < 0.05$); (iii) $- 2$ and $- 1$ ($p < 0.01$).The LH preovulatory peak is quite similar in both groups. E_2 plasma concentration in group II was rather irregular than lowered, but a severe progesterone deficiency was observed (Figure 4); due to the small number of patients, a weak statistical difference is observed only on day 6 ($p < 0.1$).

157

Clinical abnormality of prolactin secretion has been eliminated (Figure 5).

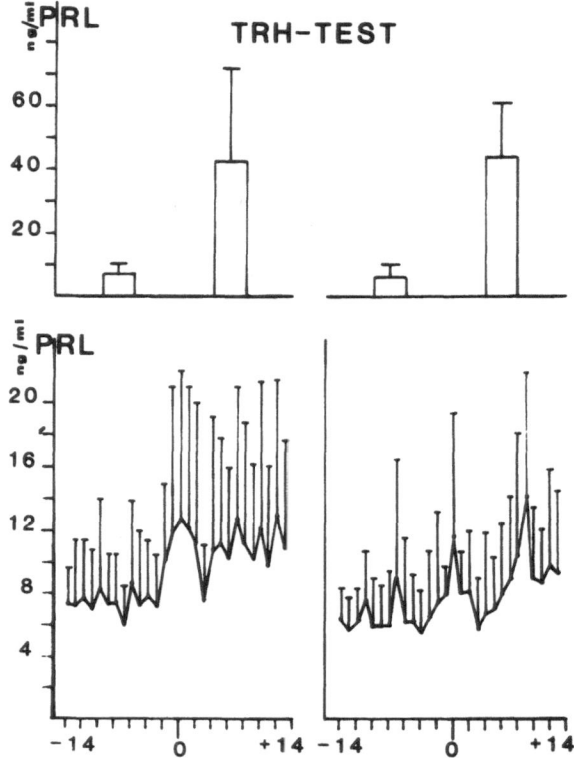

Figure 5 Clinical evaluation of prolactin (PRL) secretion in two groups of patients (group I on the left, group II on the right). An increase is noticed during the luteal phase of both groups, without any significant difference (lower panels). There is no significant difference between the results of a thyrotrophin releasing hormone (TRH) test (upper panels): basal values are on the left, on the right are peak values after 250 µg bolus of TRH

Discussion

The concept of LD was originally built on clinical observation and endometrial investigation[2–4,7]. More recently, short luteal phase has been described, which appears as a particular aspect of LD, and a striking similarity between human and monkeys has been observed[14–16]. In humans, measurements of gonadotrophins in case of luteal defect (either short or inadequate luteal phase), have already been performed, and low values of FSH have been observed[15–17]. However, these observations are scarce[18], and several patients had concomitant endocrine or metabolic disorders[17]. Then, an abnormality of gonadotrophin secretion could be suspected but not assessed by these previous results. These new data set forth both precision and confirmation.

Different studies in rhesus monkeys have demonstrated an abnormality of both FSH secretion and FSH:LH ratio patterns during the cycle[16,19,20]. LD has been induced in the rhesus monkey by specific inhibition of FSH during the first week of the cycle[15]. It can be avoided if exogenous FSH compensation is administered at the same period[22], so luteal phase dysfunction might be a sequel to abnormal folliculogenesis due to aberrant gonadotrophin secretion[23]. In our experience, this fascinating hypothesis could not be entirely confirmed in clinical practice. In most cases complementary exogenous FSH administration (Neopergonal, Searle) did not improve the BBT curve, nor the endometrial biopsy, nor the fecundity rate. In a few cases, it was followed by anovulatory cycles as if desensitization of granulosa cells had been induced. In a few other cases, the cycle was improved and pregnancy occurred (unpublished data). In human spontaneous LD, the ovarian stimulatory abnormality appears more complex than the FSH insufficiency alone. The FSH/LH balance may be more important. FSH:LH ratio should be used more frequently for clinical investigation of gynaecological disorders and/or infertility, as a low ratio would indicate FSH–LH imbalance. However, respective values of FSH and LH must be considered, and it is really interesting to notice the frequent LH rise in pituitary–ovarian dysfunction. It is quite moderate and inconstant in LD, much higher in polycystic ovarian disease. Whether it is due to an hypothalamic and/or pituitary perturbation, to a feedback insensitivity, or to an ovarian dysfunction is speculative.

These human data set forth that LD is not univocal: there are different groups of patients according to the endometrium pattern, or the FSH:LH ratio evolution. They may correspond to clinical or physiological different aspects, or both. Different and particular clinical situations are frequently associated with LD, including some forms of hyperprolactinaemia, recurrent abortions, ovulation induction[1]. This study demonstrated the possible value of FSH:LH ratio for investigation of menstrual cycle disorders, but some patients have very low FSH:LH ratio values, others have a moderate decrease of this ratio, and others only have an abnormal FSH pattern during the late follicular phase. These gonadotrophin abnormalities had already been observed in the rhesus monkey[14], but in contrast to the monkey, they are often repetitive in the human and may lead to infertility. To try to determine these different groups of patients should be a new clinical investigation challenge, towards better therapeutic methods. These results contribute to demonstrate that the endometrium is the endpoint of a cascade of hormonal influences which must be estimated by themselves and correlated together. Such a study has been attempted with prolactin.

PROLACTIN INVESTIGATION: RESPONSE TO TRH TEST

The hypothesis of a prolactin (PRL) influence on menstrual cycle disorders has been proposed, and the aim of this study is to appreciate whether it is worthwhile. The inhibiting influence of hyperprolactinaemia on cyclic gonadotrophins secretion is well documented[24–26], although its direct physiologic and/or blocking influence on the ovary is still debated, at least in primates[27, 28].

Another reason to suspect PRL influence on menstrual cycle disorders has been raised by the bromocriptine effectiveness to induce ovulation, or cure some cases of idiopathic sterility when basal prolactinaemia was in normal range[29, 30].

As PRL plasma concentration fluctuates along a 24-hour period[31, 32], and is modified by numerous circumstances ranging from stress[33] to meals[34], the thyrotrophin releasing hormone test (TRH test) has been proposed to investigate pituitary PRL secretion and possibly demonstrate inapparent functional hyperprolactinaemia[35, 36].

It has been used to investigate patients suffering gynaecological disorders with *normal basal prolactinaemia.*

Materials and methods

Patients

The patients studied ($n = 104$) were not an homogeneous population. They were complaining of different disorders, but all displayed baseline prolactin plasma levels within the normal range (< 20 ng ml^{-1}). They were subdivided into two groups according to the presence ($n = 46$) or the absence of galactorrhoea ($n = 58$) (Table 3).

Table 3 Classification of the 104 patients who were submitted to TRH test in the mid-follicular phase

	Galactorrhoea	
Investigation	With	Without
Clinical evaluation only:		
Controls	—	10
Normal cycles	16	—
Cycle disorders	10	—
Endocrine investigation:		
Luteal defects (LD)		
Pure LD	6	11
LD with oestrogenic influence	9	17
Oligomenorrhoea and amenorrhoea	5	20
Total	46	58

In the group without galactorrhoea, 10 patients were used as controls: their fecundity and the clinical aspects of their cycles were normal: they were using IUD for contraception and volunteered for the TRH test; they were not submitted to any other endocrine investigation. The other 48 patients of this group were investigated for gynaecological disorders: suspected luteal defect, oligomenorrhoea and amenorrhoea (Table 3). Among the 46 patients with galactorrhoea, 26 had only clinical evaluation, and 20 had a more precise endocrine evaluation for suspected luteal defect, oligomenorrhoea or amenorrhoea.

The ages of the patients were quite similar in the different groups (Table 4).

Table 4 Age (in years) of patients in the different groups

Group	No.	Mean ($\pm$ SE)	Range
Control	10	30.60 ± 4.84	26–41
Anovulation	25	25.20 ± 5.27	18–43
LD	17	29.23 ± 5.34	24–42
LD + PEI	26	27.88 ± 5.01	17–41
With galactorrhoea	46	29.07 ± 5.77	19–42
Without galactorrhoea	58	27.72 ± 5.26	18–43

LD = luteal defect; PEI = persistent oestrogenic influence

Endocrine evaluation

A TRH test was performed in all these 104 outpatients during the mid-follicular phase[37]. Eight blood samples were taken: two before and six after a 250 µg bolus of synthetic TRH (Stimu-TSH, Laboratoires, Roussel). Prolactin measurements used a double antibody RIA assay (CEA-Sorlin kits).

The gynaecological and endocrine investigations in 68 patients included BBT charts, endometrial biopsy, plasma steroid and gonadotrophin measurements. Except for endometrial biopsy, they will not be taken into consideration in this study. Endometrial biopsies (sampled between day 21 and 23 of the cycle) have been used in this study to classify different groups of patients.

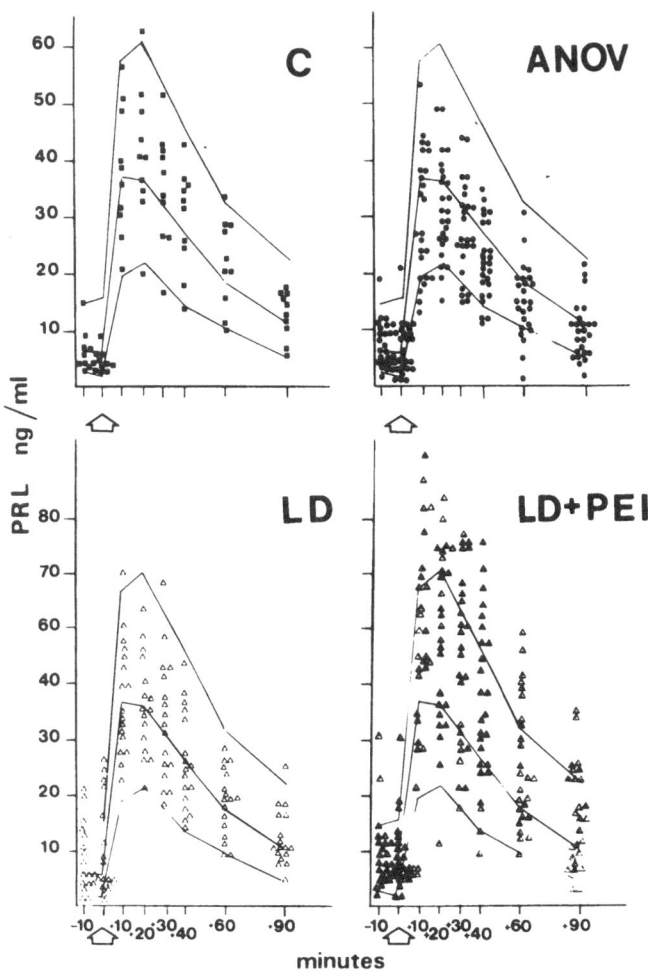

Figure 6 Prolactin values during thyrotrophin releasing hormone test in different patient groups. C = controls; ANOV = oligomenorrhoea and amenorrhoea; LD = pure luteal defect; LD + PEI = luteal defect with persistent oestrogenic influence. The lines display 10th, 50th and 90th percentiles of the whole population

Statistical methodology

TRH test—Percentiles of prolactin values were calculated.
Gynaecological and endocrine investigations—The non-parametric Wilcoxon test has been used for comparison of different parameters of the TRH test pattern: basal values, peak values, and area under the curves.

Results

Taking into consideration the PRL levels obtained in all the 104 TRH tests, in a rough comparison, percentiles were calculated, not to appreciate a standard distribution, but to display the whole of the test and set forth possible clusters of

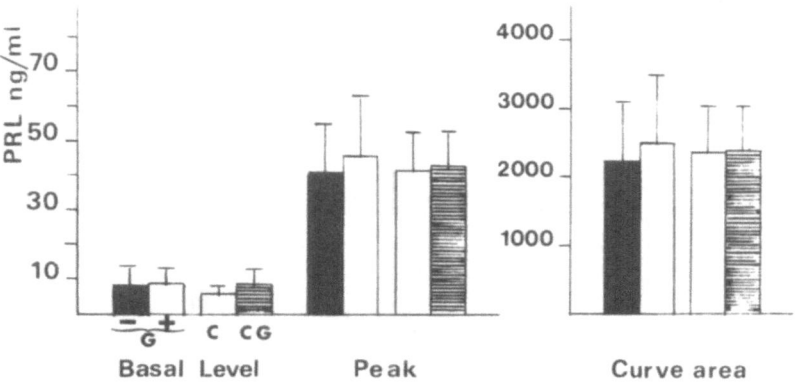

Figure 7 Comparison of prolactin (PRL) basal level, peak value and curve area, among four patient groups: with $(G+)$, without $(G-)$ galactorrhoea, and normal cycles without (C) or with (CG) galactorrhoea (see Table 5)

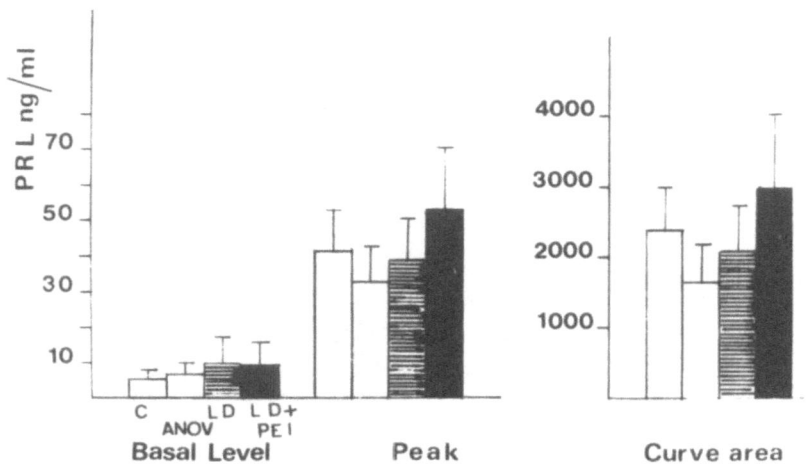

Figure 8 Comparison of prolactin (PRL) basal level, peak value and curve area, among four patient groups: C = controls; ANOV = oligomenorrhoea–amenorrhoea; luteal defect (LD) without or with persistent oestrogenic influence (PEI)

values. In each category, values were scattered. Nevertheless, this approach shows that:

(1) The 10 controls and the pure LD are distributed within percentiles 10 and 90 (Figure 6).
(2) Many values in LD + PEI are over percentile 90.
(3) Values in patients with oligomenorrhoea and amenorrhoea (ANOV) are below percentile 75.

Since the first rough descriptive study was stimulating, a more refined comparative one was undertaken. Three parameters of the TRH test curve were chosen: the PRL basal value, the zenith point (peak) and the area between the curve and the basal value. Means and standard error of means were calculated for each group and then compared using the Wilcoxon test (Table 5, Figures 7 and 8).

The 46 patients with galactorrhoea were compared with the 58 patients without galactorrhoea. No significant statistical difference was observed (Figure 7, Table 5). However, the basal level of PRL is higher in normal cycles when galactorrhoea has been observed ($p < 0.05$) (Figure 7, Table 5).

Concerning the cycle disorders observed in this population, the comparison has been estimated versus controls and between the different pathological groups themselves.

Pathological groups versus control group (Table 5, Figure 8)

The values of *basal prolactin levels* are higher in LD and LD + PEI groups. As the values are very scattered, this difference is not statistically significant. The *peak value* is significantly higher in the case of LD + PEI ($p < 0.05$), similar for LD, and lower in patients with oligomenorrhoea or amenorrhoea, without statistical significance ($p < 0.1$). The *curve area* of LD and PEI is more important but without statistical significance, that of LD is similar, that of the oligomenorrhoea–amenorrhoea group is significantly less important ($p < 0.02$).

Both types of LD versus oligomenorrhoea–amenorrhoea

Mean prolactin basal level was higher in LD and in LD + PEI but the difference was only statistically significant in the latter case ($p < 0.05$). This was also true for peak values: LD + PEI, ($p < 0.01$), LD, (NS). The curve area is increased in both luteal defect groups: $p < 0.01$ for LD and PEI, $p < 0.05$ for LD (Table 5, Figure 8).

Comparison between both groups of LD

If the baseline levels are similar, both peak value and curve area are significantly more important in LD and PEI patients: $p < 0.01$ and $p < 0.05$, respectively (Table 6, Figure 8).

Discussion

TRH is a physiological regulator of thyrotrophin secretion by the pituitary, and also stimulates PRL secretion in normal subjects[38]. It is synthesized in neurones and released from nerve terminals into the portal system, reaches the pituitary and acts directly on the pituitary cells[39]. The TRH test, inducing PRL stimulation, has already been widely used for physiological investigation[40] or evaluation of pathological situations[41].

163

Table 5 Prolactin values (as means ± SE) during TRH test in the different groups

| Value | Galactorrhoea | | Normal cycles | | ANOV (n=25) | LD (n=17) | LD and PEI (n=26) |
	Present (n=46)	Absent (n=58)	With galactorrhoea (n=16)	Controls (n=10)			
Basal level (ng ml^{-1})	8.41 ± 4.67	7.85 ± 5.84	8.31 ± 4.04	5.50 ± 2.31	6.86 ± 3.90	9.70 ± 7.46	9.36 ± 6.11
Peak value (ng ml^{-1})	45.74 ± 17.51	41.33 ± 14.56	43.37 ± 11.32	42.00 ± 11.34	33.52 ± 9.90	39.52 ± 11.13	53.73 ± 16.86
Curve area	2535.89 ± 1049.75	2260.09 ± 867.67	2419.97 ± 646.95	2379.50 ± 676.78	1783.46 ± 574.92	2227.35 ± 664.45	2962.34 ± 1076.20

ANOV = oligomenorrhoea and amenorrhoea; LD = luteal defect; PEI = persistent oestrogenic influence

If the central origin of LD is assumed, the role of PRL must be considered. It is obvious for tumoural and/or spontaneous hyperprolactinaemia. But it is debated when basal prolactinaemia is within the normal range: it has been proposed that PRL may be involved in 20% of cases of female infertility[42]. These results demonstrate that in case of LD with persistent oestrogenic influence (LD + PEI), lactotroph cells appear more responsive than usual to the TRH test: basal levels, peak values and curve areas are higher than normal. On the contrary, lactotrophs appear less responsive in case of oligomenorrhoea and amenorrhoea. A nyctemeral investigation of PRL has been performed in four of these TRH high reactive patients, and a higher sleep prolactinaemia was observed (unpublished data).

Both series of results about gonadotrophins and PRL variations in case of luteal defect stimulated us to consider more precisely menstrual cycle investigation in routine clinical practice, for a better understanding of both normal physiological patterns and functional disorders.

A RATIONALE FOR THE INVESTIGATION OF THE MENSTRUAL CYCLE

There is a wide gap between the sophisticated investigations used for the study of physiological patterns of hypothalamo-pituitary–gonadal regulations and clinical practice. On the one hand those investigations are much too time consuming and complicated, they require great co-operation from the volunteers and they cannot be performed in an outpatient clinic on people who complain of a disorder and want to be cured. On the other hand, most gynaecologists do not consider that they are facing spontaneous models, the analysis of which may suggest clues for a better understanding of correlative and/or disturbed mechanisms, by comparison with a small control group. A compromise should be defined between both these attitudes, and a more physiological concept of clinical investigation should be adopted. This physiological approach of clinical disorders may lead to a better classification of syndromes, of different groups of patients, and a better application of therapy. Such a more interrogative attitude from clinicians would facilitate fruitful exchanges with physiologists or biochemists and attainment of new concepts for physiopathology and therapy. Two recent examples of this type of physiological clinical research can be set forth: the importance of gonadotrophin pulsatility and, in our opinion, LD.

A method of investigation of the menstrual cycle has been devised. It is easily acceptable by patients, while taking account of the information described before. It applies essentially to ovulatory cycles. Its preliminary results appear to demonstrate that the physiopathology of LD is not univocal, and that there may be several different groups of patients.

Investigation methodology (Figure 9)

The BBT curve is, of course, the beginning of this investigation. The ovulation is presumed, and lengths of both follicular and luteal phases are estimated in days[7].

During the follicular phase

As the influence of FSH, LH, and the value of FSH:LH ratio appear to be essential during the first week of the menstrual cycle, the investigation begins on the first or second day of the cycle: three measurements of plasma FSH and LH are performed either on days 1, 3 and 5, or 2, 4 and 6. The FSH:LH ratio is calculated on each daily sample. Oestradiol-17β is measured in each sample and testosterone and Δ_4-androstenedione are evaluated once during the same period.

To appreciate a normal PRL secretion or, on the contrary, an unsuspected hyperprolactinaemia, a TRH test is performed between days 9 and 12, at the beginning of the late follicular phase.

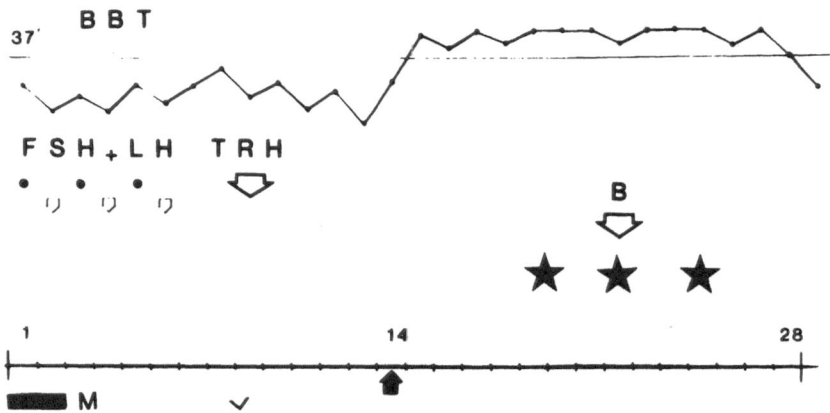

Figure 9 Proposed method of investigation of the menstrual cycle disorders. BBT = basal body temperature; M = menstruation; B = endometrial biopsy

During the luteal phase

An endometrial biopsy was performed on days 22 or 23, and three measurements of plasma oestradiol and progesterone on days 19, 22 and 25 were taken.

Such an investigation leads to a bioclinical survey of the whole menstrual cycle. The comparison of these results with normal cycle data at the same periods may give information on the biological aspects and determinants of clinical disorders.

Preliminary results

This investigation has been performed on 52 patients. Data concerning FSH, LH and PRL will only be discussed here according to clinical and endometrial situations.

The mean ($\pm$ SE) value of FSH:LH ratio of 27 normal cycles has been calculated for each day, the cycles being synchronized from the LH peak. Those values from day -14 to day -7 have been used for comparison with those observed during the first week of the cycle in different clinical situations (Figure 10). Obviously, in case of LD + PEI and anovulation, the mean value of FSH:LH ratio is low.

If the PRL peak during the TRH test is considered, values are more scattered (Figure 11). The comparison is less conclusive, but the diagram is very similar to that in Figure 6, with a low response in the anovulation group.

Table 6 Mean ($\pm$ SE) FSH:LH ratios, prolactin (PRL) basal and peak values in 52 patients distributed in four groups, according to endometrium pattern

Hormone	Endometrium			
	Normal (n = 6)	Luteal defect (n = 16)	Luteal defect with PEI (n = 19)	Anovulation (n = 11)
FSH:LH	1.95 ± 0.84	1.73 ± 0.33	1.37 ± 0.71	1.18 ± 0.49
PRL (ng ml^{-1}):				
Basal level	7.25 ± 4.08	6.75 ± 4.34	9.29 ± 5.12	6.09 ± 3.06
Peak value	52.17 ± 14.40	49.31 ± 18.82	50.68 ± 21.46	34.45 ± 16.75

PEI = persistent oestrogenic influence

167

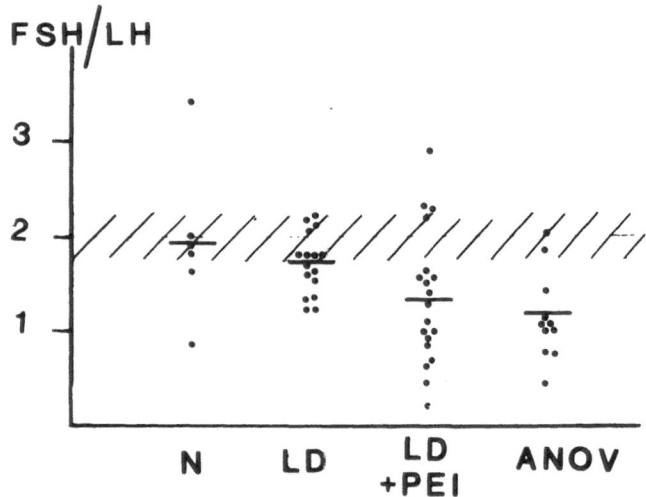

Figure 10 FSH:LH ratio in different clinical situations. The hatched area represents the means and SE of 27 normal cycles from day -14 to day -7. The individual values of different groups of patients are plotted: normal patients (N), those with luteal defect (LD), luteal defect and persistent oestrogenic influence (LD + PEI), and those with anovulatory cycles (ANOV). Means are given as solid lines (see Table 6)

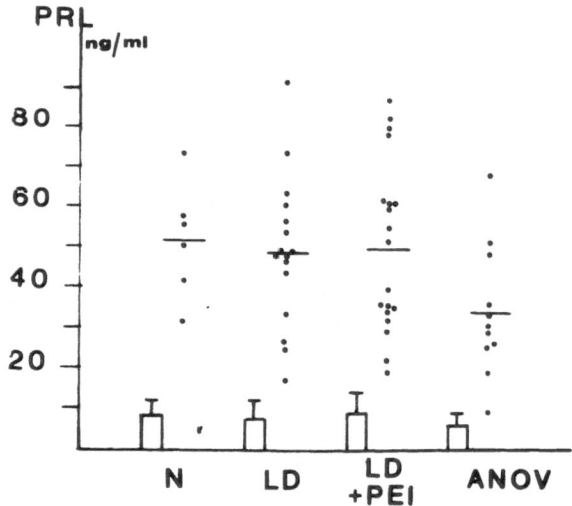

Figure 11 Mean ($\pm$ SE) prolactin (PRL) basal values in different groups of patients (columns); peak PRL values and their means in the same patients are shown as dots and solid lines, respectively. Abbreviations as in Figure 10 (see Table 6)

Comments

This preliminary investigation demonstrates that it becomes easier to understand the biological patterns of clinical disorders. *Anovulation* is characterized by an imbalanced secretion and/or reactivity of both gonadotroph and lactotroph cells; whether it is due to an insufficient hypothalamic stimulation or to the cell inability remains to be ascertained. *Pure LD* appears as biologically near from normal: it may be a transient spontaneously regressive or easy to cure perturbation. *LD plus persistent oestrogenic influence* appears to deserve a peculiar specificity:

(1) High frequency of delayed ovulation.
(2) Specific endometrial patterns.
(3) Important abnormalities of ovarian steroid secretions[5].
(4) Anomalies of FSH, LH and sometimes of PRL secretion. In our experience LD + PEI appears more recurrent and more difficult to improve than pure LD.

However, this better understanding of biological pattern demonstrates that patients with clinically similar disorders may have different endocrine perturbations. For instance, patients with LD + PEI may have low or high TRH responsitivity. Such peculiar biological aspects may have a therapeutic effect: for instance, a dopaminergic anti-PRL therapy may be chosen in some cases with a better information.

Such a bioclinical approach should enlighten the physiopathology of clinical situations. These results rather conflict with those reported by Peillon *et al.*[36]. The interpretation of these authors may be somewhat superficial.

In conclusion, it is highly probable that such aspects of clinical physiology will lead to a better characterization of clinical syndromes, to a better gathering of patients, or better therapeutic choices, and using these spontaneous physiopathological models, to a better approach of endocrine regulations.

References

1. Wentz, A. C. (1982). Diagnosing luteal phase inadequacy. *Fertil. Steril.*, **37**, 334–5
2. Jones, G. S. (1949). Some newer aspects of the management of infertility. *J. Am. Med. Assoc.*, **141**, 1123
3. Moszkowski, E., Woodruff, J. D. and Jones, G. S. (1962). The inadequate luteal phase. *Am. J. Obstet. Gynecol.*, **83**, 363–9
4. Jones, G. S. (1976). The luteal phase defect. *Fertil. Steril.*, **27**, 351–6
5. Gautray, J. P., de Brux, J., Tajchner, G., Robel, P. and Mouren, M. (1981). Clinical investigation of the menstrual cycle. III. Clinical, endometrial and endocrine aspects of luteal defect. *Fertil. Steril.*, **35**, 296–303
6. Wentz, A. C. (1982). Physiologic and clinical considerations in luteal phase defect. *Clin. Obstet. Gynecol.*, **22**, 169–85
7. Jolivet, A. and Gautray, J. P. (1978). Clinical investigation of the menstrual cycle. I. Diagram of the normal menstrual cycle. *Fertil. Steril.*, **29**, 40–3
8. de Brux, J. (1981). Evaluation of ovarian disturbances by endometrial biopsy. In de Brux, J., Mortel, R., and Gautray, J. P. (eds.) *The Endometrium: Hormonal Impacts.* Vol. 1, pp. 107–220. (New York: Plenum Press)
9. Daly, D. C., Tohan, N., Doney, T. J., Maslar, I. A. and Riddick, D. H. (1982). The significance of lymphocytic–leukocytic infiltrates in interpreting late luteal phase endometrial biopsies. *Fertil. Steril.*, **87**, 786–91
10. Castanier, M. and Scholler, R. (1970). Dosage radio-immunologique de l'estrone et de l'estradiol 17 beta plasmatiques. *C. R. Acad. Sci. (Paris)*, **271**, 1787–9
11. Roger, M., Veinante, A., Soldat, M. C., Tardy, J., Tribondeau, E. and Scholler, R. (1975). Etude simultanée des gonadotrophines, des oestrogènes, de la progestérone, et de la 17-hydroxy progestérone plasmatiques au cours du cycle ovulatoire. *N. Press. Med.*, **4**, 2173–8
12. Tea, N. T., Castanier, M., Roger, M. and Scholler, R. (1975). Simultaneous radio-immunoassay of plasma progesterone, and 17-hydroxyprogesterone. Normal values in children, in men, and in women throughout the menstrual cycle and in early pregnancy. *J. Steroid Biochem.*, **6**, 1509–16
13. Lebard, L. (1970). *Traitement des Données Statistiques.* Vol. 1, pp. 384–7. (Paris: Dunod)
14. Strott, C. A., Cargille, C. M., Ross, G. T. and Lipsett, M. B. (1970). The short luteal phase. *J. Clin. Endocrinol. Metab.*, **30**, 246–52

15. Sherman, B. M. and Korenman, S. G. (1974). Measurement of plasma LH, FSH, estradiol and progesterone in disorders of the human menstrual cycle: the short luteal phase. *J. Clin. Endocrinol. Metab.*, **38**, 89–93

16. Nass, T. E., Dierschke, D. J., Clerk, J. R., Meller, P. A. and Schillo, K. K. (1979). Luteal phase deficiencies in peripubertal rhesus monkeys: mechanistic considerations. In Channing, C. P., Marsh, J. and Sadler, W. A. (eds.) *Ovarian Follicular and Corpus Luteum Function.* pp. 519–25. (New York: Plenum Press)

17. Sherman, B. M. and Korenman, S. G. (1974). Measurement of serum LH, FSH, estradiol and progesterone in disorders of the human menstrual cycle: the inadequate luteal phase. *J. Clin. Endocrinol. Metab.*, **39**, 145–9

18. Aksel, S. (1980). Sporadic and recurrent luteal phase defect in cyclic women: comparison with normal cycles. *Fertil. Steril.*, **33**, 372–7

19. Wilks, J. W., Hodgen, G. D. and Ross, G. T. (1976). Luteal phase defects in the rhesus monkey: the significance of serum FSH:LH ratios. *J. Clin. Endocrinol. Metab.*, **43**, 1261–7

20. Wilks, J. W., Hodgen, G. D. and Ross, G. T. (1977). Anovulatory menstrual cycles in the rhesus monkey: the significance of serum FSH/LH ratios. *Fertil. Steril.*, **28**, 1094–1100

21. Stouffer, R. L. and Hodgen, G. D. (1980). Induction of luteal phase defects in rhesus monkey by follicular fluid administration at the onset of the menstrual cycle. *J. Clin. Endocrinol. Metab.*, **51**, 669–71

22. Dizerega, G. S. and Hodgen, G. D. (1981). Follicular phase treatment of luteal phase dysfunction. *Fertil. Steril.*, **35**, 489–99

23. Dizerega, G. S. and Hodgen, G. D. (1981). Luteal phase dysfunction infertility: a sequel to aberrant folliculogenesis. *Fertil. Steril.*, **35**, 489–99

24. Tyson, J. E., Khojandi, M., Huth, J., Smith, B. and Thomas, P. (1975). Inhibition of cyclic gonadotropin secretion by endogenous human prolactin. *Am. J. Obstet. Gynecol.*, **121**, 375

25. Lachelin, G. C. L., Abu-Fadil, S. and Yen, S. S. C. (1977). Functional delineation of hyperprolactinemic amenorrhea. *J. Clin. Endocrinol. Metab.*, **44**, 1163

26. Besser, G. M. (1982). Interaction between the mechanisms controlling prolactin and gonadotrophin secretion. In Clauser, H. and Gautray, J. P. (eds.) *Prolactine, Neurotransmission et Fertilité.* Vol. 1, pp. 209–17. (Paris: Masson)

27. Balmaceda, J. P., Eddy, C. A., Smith, C. G. and Asch, R. H. (1981). The effects of hyperprolactinemia on the luteal phase of the rhesus monkey: evidence for a direct prolactin effect on the ovary. American Fertility Society Meeting. *Fertil. Steril.*, **36**, 431

28. McNeilly, A. S. (1982). Prolactin and the control of ovarian function. In Clauser, H. and Gautray, J. P. (eds.) *Prolactine, Neurotransmission et Fertilité.* Vol. 1, pp. 1–8. (Paris: Masson)

29. Tolis, G. and Naftolin, F. (1976). Induction of menstruation with bromocryptine in patients with euprolactinaemic amenorrhea. *Am. J. Obstet. Gynecol.*, **126**, 426–31

30. Koike, K., Aono, T., Miyake, A., Tsutsumi, H., Matsumoto, K. and Kurachi, K. (1981). Induction of ovulation in patients with normoprolactinemic amenorrhea by combined therapy with bromocriptine and clomiphene. *Fertil. Steril.*, **35**, 138–41

31. Sassin, J., Frantz, A., Weitzman, E. and Kapen, S. (1972). Human prolactin: 24-hour pattern with increased release during sleep. *Science*, **177**, 1205

32. Polleri, D., Barreca, T., Cicchetti, V., Gianrossi, R., Masturzo, P. and Rolandi, R. (1976). The 24th pattern of human prolactin in serum. *Chronobiologia*, **3**, 27

33. Hagen, C., Brandt, M. R. and Kehlet, H. (1980). Prolactin, LH, FSH, GH and cortisol response to surgery and the effect of epidural analgesia. *Acta Endocrinol.*, **94**, 151–4

34. Quigley, M. E., Ropert, J. F. and Yen, S. S. C. (1981). Acute prolactin release triggered by feeding. *J. Clin. Endocrinol. Metab.*, **52**, 1043–6

35. Perez-Lopez, F. R., Gomez Agudo, G. and Abos, M. D. (1981). Serum prolactin and thyrotrophin responses to TRH at different times of the day in normal women. *Acta Endocrinol.*, **97**, 7–11

36. Peillon, F., Vincens, M., Cesselin, F., Doumith, R. and Mowszowicz, I. (1982). Exaggerated prolactin response of TRH in women with anovulatory cycles: possible role of endogenous estrogens and effect of bromocriptine. *Fertil. Steril.*, **37**, 530–5

37. Vekemans, M., Delvove, P., l'Hermite, M. and Robyn, C. (1977). Serum prolactin levels during the menstrual cycle. *J. Clin. Endocrinol. Metab.*, **44**, 989–93

38. Enjalbert, A. (1982). Multiple factors which influence prolactin secretion by the pituitary. In Clauser, H. and Gautray, J. P. (eds.) *Prolactin, Neurotransmission and Fertility.* Vol 1, pp. 75–96. (Paris: Masson)

39. Prange, A. J. and Utiger, R. D. (1981). What does brain thyrotropin releasing hormone do? *N. Engl. J. Med.*, **305**, 1089–90

40. Djursing, H., Hagen, C., Moller, J. and Christiansen, C. (1981). Short and long term fluctuations in plasma prolactin concentration in normal subjects. *Acta Endocrinol.*, **97**, 1–6
41. Assies, J., Schellekens, A. P. M. and Touber, J. L. (1980). The value of an intravenous TRH test for the diagnosis of tumoral prolactinemia. *Acta Endocrinol.*, **94**, 439–49
42. Kedentser, J. V., Hoskins, C. F. and Scott, J. Z. (1981). Hyperprolactinemia. A significant factor in female infertility. *Am. J. Obstet. Gynecol.*, **139**, 264–7

12
Gonadotrophin-resistant ovaries: a desensitization syndrome?

A. P. Netter and A. E. Lambert

Insensitivity to protein hormones can be due to a variety of mechanisms. In the human, ovarian resistance to PMSG has been known for a long time: it is related to the development of *antibodies* to this foreign protein.

An example of *anti-receptor* antibodies occurs in *myasthenia gravis*, a disease due to the presence of antibodies against the acetylcholine receptor[1].

No such antibodies have been detected in the gonadotrophin-resistant ovary syndrome (GROS). The aims of this chapter are:

(1) To demonstrate that GROS is a relatively common disease.
(2) To study its aetiology.
(3) To show that oestrogen treatment can result in the recovery of ovarian function.
(4) To suggest that GROS could be a desensitization syndrome of the ovarian gonadotrophin receptors.

A COMMON DISEASE

According to G. S. Jones and M. de Moraes Ruehsen[2], GROS is characterized by the association of primary amenorrhoea, normal development of secondary sexual characteristics, elevated urinary gonadotrophins, the presence of many primordial follicles in the ovaries and the absence of an ovarian response to stimulation by human gonadotrophins.

Twelve years earlier[3], we had reported 10 cases of what we called '*ovarioplegic amenorrhoea*', the characteristics of which were identical, except that in our cases amenorrhoea was secondary and not primary.

Since then, numerous cases of GROS with secondary amenorrhoea have been reported[4–7].

When one looks at Jones' cases again, one finds clear evidence of ovarian function over several months—despite the primary amenorrhoea—in the normal development of the mammary glands. The important feature of the syndrome in a young woman is the presence of *hypergonadotrophic amenorrhoea with the persistence of ovarian follicles*.

AETIOLOGY

GROS can be observed in many circumstances. It should first be noted that during the several months or years preceding the *menopause* (the peri- or pre-menopause), there are intervals of amenorrhoea with hot flushes, elevated urinary and plasma gonadotrophins and insensitivity to stimulation with hMG.

The ovary becomes less sensitive to exogenous stimulation with advancing age; induction of ovulation requires higher doses of hMG during the fourth decade of life than during the third decade, as we showed in 1965.

Sufficiently powerful doses of *roentgentherapy* and *antimitotic* drugs can induce temporary, but long-lasting, amenorrhoea, with all the characteristics of GROS.

The same is true for extensive *surgical resection* of the ovary removing more than four-fifths of the ovarian parenchyma.

Psychogenic GROS is exemplified by the cases which our group published in 1957[3], but also by the cases summed up in Table 1.

Table 1 Psychogenic GROS. In the six cases reported here, FSH and LH were constantly at the post-menopausal level

Case	Age at first examination	Amenorrhoea began at	Immediately after	Follicles in ovarian biopsy
1	20	14 after oligo	Divorce of parents	Primary
2	18	17	Divorce of parents and first intercourse	Primary and antral
3	22	20 after oligo	Rape	
4	22	19 sudden	Remarriage of mother	Primary and antral
5	36	33 after oligo	Abandoned by husband	Primary
6	26	22 sudden	Suicide of mother	Primary

Amenorrhoea is secondary in many cases of *ovarian dysgenesis*. Pregnancy is a rare event, but 10 babies have been born to Turnerian mothers.

The evolution of some cases of mild ovarian dysgenesis has been followed by laparoscopy and ovarian biopsy[8]. Small, elongated, follicle-containing ovaries eventually became *streak* gonads made up solely of fibrous connective tissue. In her first case, Jones speaks of 'fat streak ovaries'[2]. No doubt a few years later, these ovaries had become transformed into streak gonads, devoid of any follicles.

The final and most interesting category comprises the cases of *idiopathic* GROS where, not only is there no chromosomal anomaly, but also the ovaries are of normal adult size and shape and contain innumerable follicles, as shown in Figure 1. In a peculiar variant of idiopathic GROS, amenorrhoea is intermittent: periods of normal menstruation with normal gonadotrophin levels alternate with periods of amenorrhoea with high gonadotrophins. Pregnancy can occur during a normal phase of this intermittent disease. Such a case was observed recently in a 29-year-old woman who presented with phases of amenorrhoea with plasma FSH levels varying between 19 mIU/ml and 28 mIU/ml, LH levels between 14 and 18 mIU/ml, and E_2 levels between 20 and 30 pg/ml. Her karyotype was normal. During rest-periods and vacations, 4–5 normal cycles appeared. Amenorrhoea recurred as soon as she became emotionally upset, particularly in her work.

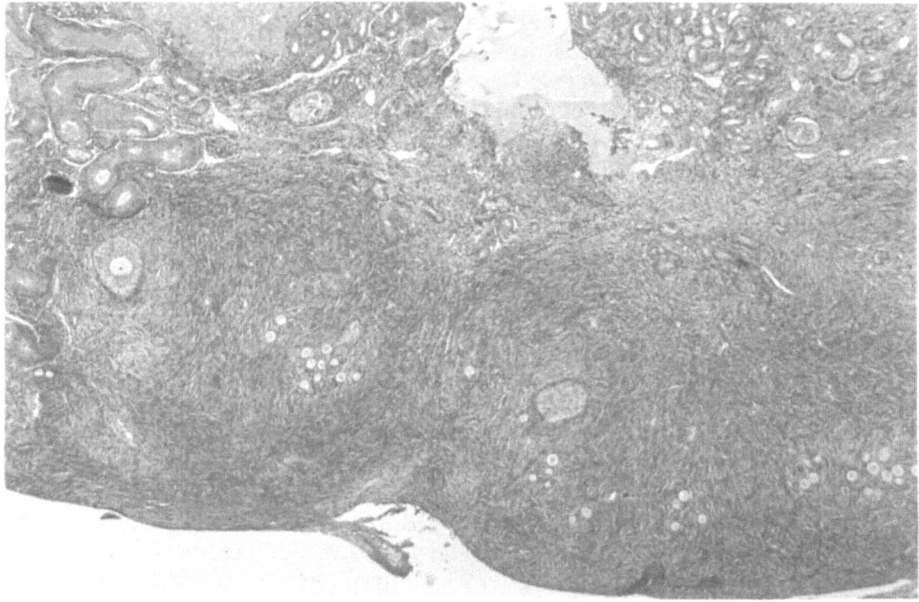

Figure 1 GROS: microscopic appearance of the ovary in one of our cases. A number of follicles of various sizes and degrees of development can be seen

THE EFFECTS OF OESTROGEN TREATMENT

The effects are illustrated by the following case.

Mrs A, aged 26, from Morocco, presented with primary amenorrhoea and sterility. She had been married 7 years. She arrived with a fairly complete medical history behind her, having been examined and investigated at 17. At that time, a diagnosis of gonadal dysgenesis had been made on the basis of the following results:

(1) The level of total urinary gonadotrophins was 40–80 mu.
(2) The karyotype was 46XX/45X0.
(3) The ovarian biopsy performed through laparotomy reported 'a uterus the size of an almond, tubes 1 mm thick, with rudimentary ostia, and ovaries the size and appearance of a date pit, 25 × 10 mm'. The biopsy showed primary follicles, and no antral follicles.

She had been treated with sequential oestrogens and progestogens, which had resulted in the development of normal secondary sexual characteristics.

When we first examined her, she had been under no therapy for a year. She was an attractive young woman, of normal height (1.6 m), and with well-developed pubic and axillary hair, and normal breasts. The fourth metacarpal was slightly short, and she had no other somatic abnormality. Vulva, vagina and uterus were hypoplastic. Hysterography revealed a small hypoplastic and slightly arcuate uterus. The tubes were patent. Plasma FSH level was 35 mIU (normal range at that age: 2–5 mIU), LH level was 27 mIU (normal: 1.5–3 mIU) and oestradiol level was 10 pg/ml.

At laparoscopy we noted a streak gonad on the right; the appearance of the left ovary was almost the same as that described 9 years earlier. No biopsy was performed on account of the small size of this unilateral rudimentary ovary.

To sum up: this was a case of primary amenorrhoea and sterility obviously due to gonadal dysgenesis in a white 46XX/45X0 female.

Although the functional prognosis seemed desperate, we planned to try to induce ovulation after prolonged treatment with sequential steroid cycles. This was prescribed because we have on our files a few cases of gonadotrophin-resistant ovaries in which ovulation occurred spontaneously in the course of, or after, this type of prolonged artificial cycle therapy; and also because the patient had recently been unsuccessfully treated with very high doses of hMG.

After 7 months of such therapy, we tried to induce ovulation. Every day for 6 days, the patient was given eight ampoules of hMG (75U.FSH IRP 2) (600U. FSH IRP 2). On day 7, examination revealed a small amount of cervical mucus, which we scored 0.5 (scale, 0–3). Plasma oestradiol value was 54 pg/ml. She received no treatment that day, as we awaited the results of her plasma and urinary hormone investigations.

On days 8, 10, 11, 12 and 13 she received a further eight ampoules daily of hMG and 10 000 IU hCG on days 12 and 14. Basal body temperature rose on day 14 and plateaued for 25 days, after which the patient menstruated. Hormone assays gave the results shown in Table 2.

Table 2

Day of therapy	8th	9th	13th	23rd
Urinary total oestrogens (μg/24 h)	25		75	390
Urinary pregnanediol (mg/24 h)				75
Plasma oestradiol (pg/ml)		54		
Therapy: hMG 8 ampoules per day, days 1 to 6 and 8 to 12	hCG 5000 IU 12th, 14th, 17th days			

The patient then returned to Morocco, where she followed exactly the same treatment, our advice being given by telephone, though unfortunately without the help of hormone assays.

She ovulated during the next two treatment cycles and became pregnant in the third. She delivered prematurely at 6 months; the fetus was apparently normal but did not survive.

Similarly successful oestrogen therapy in idiopathic GROS has been reported[4,6].

Oestrogen therapy can be administered according to the pattern used in the above case, or in very low but continuous doses allowing ovulation to occur during treatment, as in Brosens' case and in several of our own.

Their mechanism of action is very controversial: Pencharz[14] demonstrated that in the rat, oestrogens increase the ovarian response to gonadotrophins.

Netter reported that in the human, high doses of oestrogens inhibit, and low doses enhance, the ovarian response to gonadotrophins[9]. Goldenberg found that the injection of hypophysectomized rats with DES increased the ovarian consumption of radioactive thymidine and FSH[15].

In conjunction with Pasqualini and Paniel, our own group has found (unpublished data) oestrogen receptors in human ovarian vessels, suggesting that exogenous oestrogens could play a role in revascularizing the ovaries and thus facilitating their return to normal function.

Direct oestrogen action on granulosa cells is convincingly shown by the following findings: oestrogens increase the number of granulosa cells, not the number of binding sites per cell[10]; furthermore, oestradiol enhances FSH-dependent cAMP accumulation *in vivo* and *in vitro*, in the absence of any change in the number of FSH binding sites[11].

DESENSITIZATION

Desensitization to protein hormones was first described by Gavin[12] in insulin-resistant diabetes.

Ovarian desensitization has been achieved by Richards and Jonassen in hypophysectomized rats[13]. It is easier to desensitize thecal cells to hCG than granulosa cells to FSH.

The phenomenon of desensitization would be clarified by a better understanding of how peptide hormones produce chemical signals that bring about alterations in cell metabolism.

Since Sutherland's discovery of cAMP as the second messenger for glucagon, it has been considered likely that all hormone responses using peptide messengers are attributable solely to hormone binding to the outer membrane surface and the subsequent production of a transmembrane signal. Things are not so simple, however. It is now clear that peptide hormones are internalized in their target cells through endocytic processes mediated by their specific receptors. Specific binding sites for peptide hormones seem to exist inside the receptor cell, perhaps including the nucleus.

Is there any way of demonstrating, in women with GROS, that this is a syndrome of desensitization affecting the follicular cells of the ovary? Could, for instance, any interpretable anomalies be demonstrated by transmission electron microscopy of rough endoplasmic reticulum, Golgi apparatus and lysosomes? Might it not be reasonable to make a comparative study of the fate of radioiodine- or ferritin-labelled FSH in normal and gonadotrophin-resistant women, by ultracentrifuge separation of the various cell organelles obtained in ovarian biopsy?

Whatever the mechanism of desensitization, it seems reasonable to postulate that oestrogen treatment acts through three synergistic mechanisms:

(1) Vasodilatation of the ovarian arteries and re-establishment of the ovarian circulation impaired by lack of oestrogen secretion.

(2) Direct action on the number and receptivity of granulosa cells and on the receptivity of thecal cells.

(3) Decrease in FSH and LH levels, breaking the vicious circle maintaining desensitization through the constant pressure exerted by these high levels on the FSH and LH receptors.

Returning now to clinical considerations, we report two cases that seem to support our hypothesis.

Mrs R, aged 35, had been operated upon 1 year previously for bilateral ovarian cysts: four-fifths of the ovarian parenchyma had been removed. She sought advice because, 1 year post-operatively, she had ceased menstruating and was suffering from frequent hot flushes. Plasma FSH value varied between 20 and 25 mIU/ml and E_2 value between 20 pg/ml and undetectably low levels. Ten ampoules of hMG daily for 10 days had no effect on plasma oestradiol levels. Oestrogens were then administered (ethinyloestradiol, 25 µg daily). A rise in body temperature occurred 10 days later, plasma oestradiol levels increased to 50 pg/ml and progesterone levels were 7 ng/ml. The corpus luteum lasted for only 6 days, and menstruation followed. We continued to administer ethinyloestradiol and we assayed plasma oestradiol once a week to know when we could try to stimulate the ovaries to obtain a pregnancy. When E_2 reached 75 pg/ml, 12 ampoules of hMG were injected daily for 3 days: on the fourth day, E_2 fell to non-detectable levels.

Mrs H, aged 38, had menstruated thrice yearly for 3 years, with plasma FSH levels ranging between 25 and 40 mIU/ml. Between menstruations, she suffered hot flushes and her E_2 levels varied from 20 to 35 pg/ml. She received 14 ampoules hMG daily, to no effect. Ethinyloestradiol, 25 µg daily, was prescribed on a permanent basis. When the plasma E_2 reached 60 pg/ml, 14 ampoules of hMG were injected daily for 3 days; the cycle stopped abruptly, and E_2 levels fell to 10 pg/ml. This experiment was carried out four times over 18 months, with the same result.

This would seem to suggest that without wishing to do so we may have blocked the ovarian gonadotrophin receptors. Such are the facts, but their interpretation is open to doubt. LHRH is known to block LHRH receptors in the human. Perhaps we are dealing here with a similar phenomenon and that at least is why we have reported the case histories above.

References

1. Aharonov, A., Abramsky, O., et al. (1975). Humoral antibodies to acetylcholine receptor in patients with myasthenia gravis. Lancet, 2, 340–2
2. Jones, G. S. and de Moraes-Ruehsen, M. (1969). A new syndrome of amenorrhea in association with hypergonadotropism and apparently normal ovarian follicular apparatus. Am. J. Obstet. Gynecol., 104, 597–600
3. Netter, A., Lambert, A., Lumbroso, P., Mantel, O. and Faure (1957). Aménorrhées ovario-plégiques (ménopauses neurogènes). Ann. Endocrinol., 18, 1014–20
4. Brosens, I. A., Koninckx, Ph. and Vlaemynck, G. (1979). Recovery of ovarian function in persistent hypergonadotropic state following low dose estrogen treatment. Infertility, 2, 219–26
5. Kim, M. H. (1974). 'Gonadotropin resistant ovaries' syndrome in association with secondary amenorrhea. Am. J. Obstet. Gynecol., 120, 257–62
6. Koninckx, P. R. and Brosens, I. A. (1977). The gonadotropin resistant ovary syndrome as a cause of secondary amenorrhea and infertility. Fertil. Steril., 28, 926–31
7. Starup, J., Selë, V. and Henriksen, B. (1971). Amenorrhea associated with increased production of gonadotropins and a morphologically normal ovarian follicular apparatus. Acta Endocrinol., 66, 248–56

8. Adjiman, M. (1966). *Contribution à l'Étude des Ménopauses Précoces*. PhD Thesis, University of Paris.
9. Netter, A., Lambert, A. and Rainer, S. (1966). Etude des effets des oestrogènes sur la secrétion des ovaires humains. *Rev. Eur. Endocrinol.*, **3**, 199–209
10. Louvet, J. P. and Vaitukaitis, J. L. (1976). Induction of FSH receptors in rat ovaries by oestrogen priming. *Endocrinology*, **99**, 758–64
11. Richards, J. S., Jonassen, J. A., Rolfes, A. I., Kersey, K. and Reichert, K. E. (1979). A.M.P., Luteinizing Hormone Receptor and progesterone during granulosa cell differentiation: effects of estradiol and follicle stimulating hormone. *Endocrinology*, **104**, 765–73
12. Archer, J. A., Gorden, P., Gavin, J. R., *et al.* (1973). Insulin receptors in human circulating lymphocytes. *J. Clin. Endocrinol. Metab.*, **36**, 627–39
13. Jonassen, J. A. and Richards, J. A. (1980). Granulosa cell desensitization: effects of gonadotropins on antral and preantral follicles. *Endocrinology*, **106**, 1786–94
14. Pencharz, R. I. (1940). *Science*, **91**, 954
15. Goldenberg, R. L., Vaitukaitis, J. L. and Ross, G. T. (1972). *Endocrinology*, **90**, 1492

Index